The Women's Guide to Ending Pain

An 8-Step Program

Howard S. Smith, M.D.
Debra Fulghum Bruce, M.S.

WILEY

John Wiley & Sons, Inc.

Published by John Wiley & Sons, Inc., Hoboken, New Jersey
Published simultaneously in Canada

No part of this publication may be reproduced, stored in a retrieval system, or transmitted in any form or by any means, electronic, mechanical, photocopying, recording, scanning, or otherwise, except as permitted under Section 107 or 108 of the 1976 United States Copyright Act, without either the prior written permission of the Publisher, or authorization through payment of the appropriate per-copy fee to the Copyright Clearance Center, 222 Rosewood Drive, Danvers, MA 01923, (978) 750–8400, fax (978) 750–4470, or on the web at www.copyright.com. Requests to the Publisher for permission should be addressed to the Permissions Department, John Wiley & Sons, Inc., 111 River Street, Hoboken, NJ 07030, (201) 748–6011, fax (201) 748–6008, email: permcoordinator@wiley.com.

Limit of Liability/Disclaimer of Warranty: While the publisher and the author have used their best efforts in preparing this book, they make no representations or warranties with respect to the accuracy or completeness of the contents of this book and specifically disclaim any implied warranties of merchantability or fitness for a particular purpose. No warranty may be created or extended by sales representatives or written sales materials. The advice and strategies contained herein may not be suitable for your situation. You should consult with a professional where appropriate. Neither the publisher nor the author shall be liable for any loss of profit or any other commercial damages, including but not limited to special, incidental, consequential, or other damages.

For general information about our other products and services, please contact our Customer Care Department within the United States at (800) 762–2974, outside the United States at (317) 572–3993 or fax (317) 572–4002.

Wiley also publishes its books in a variety of electronic formats. Some content that appears in print may not be available in electronic books. For more information about Wiley products, visit our web site at www.wiley.com.

To protect their privacy, pseudonyms have been used for the individual patients and case stories mentioned in this book.

Library of Congress Cataloging-in-Publication Data:
Smith, Howard S., date.
    The women's guide to ending pain : an 8-step program to treating pain / Howard S. Smith, Debra Fulghum Bruce.
       p. ; cm
Includes bibliograpical references and index.
    ISBN 0–471–26605–1 (pbk.)
    1. Chronic pain—Popular works. 2. Women—Diseases—Popular works.
3. Chronic pain—Alternate treatment—Popular works.
    [DNLM: 1. Pain—diagnosis—Popular Works. 2. Pain—therapy—Popular Works. 3. Women's Health—Popular Works. WL 704 S649w 2003] I. Bruce, Debra Fulghum, 1951- II. Title.
    RB127 .S627 2003
    616.0472'082—dc21   2002153127
Printed in the United States of America
10 9 8 7 6 5 4 3 2 1

In loving memory of my mother, Arlene
To my wife, Joan
To my children, Alyssa, Joshua, Benjamin, and Eric
—Howard Smith, M.D.

To my husband and best friend, Bob
To our children, Rob, Claire, Britt, Mike, and Ashley
To our first grandchild, Zoe
—Debra Fulghum Bruce, M.S.

Contents

Preface

I've written this book to help you get in control of chronic pain. No matter what type of pain you have or how long you have suffered, I believe that you can find effective treatment that meets your needs and finally get relief for the pain that has literally stolen your life.

Whether you experience discomfort from menstrual cramps, migraine headaches, joint pain, or the deep muscle pain of fibromyalgia, it's so easy to feel lost, overwhelmed, and beaten by chronic pain. After all, chronic pain greets you as you awaken in the morning. It reminds you of its existence throughout the day, holding you back from taking care of your family, being productive at work, and exercising or doing other activities that you enjoy. Chronic pain is there when you pull back your covers for bed; its nagging signals keep you from sleeping soundly. Moreover, as you have probably experienced, chronic pain can make women who are normally happy, energetic, and free spirited feel miserable and limited in all they do.

Most women experience pain at some time in their lives, and pain does not easily go away on its own. The statistics are startling:

- More than 130 million Americans suffer with chronic pain, and more than half of these are women.
- Pain with PMS affects about 70 to 90 percent of women during their childbearing years. About 30 to 40 percent of these women have pain symptoms severe enough to disturb the

routine of their daily life, and about 7 to 10 percent have such severe pain that it is considered disabling.

- Migraines affect 18 percent of all women. Of all headache pain experienced, 90 percent is from tension headaches.
- Four out of five women experience back pain, and 80 percent of these have it for more than one year. Women's back pain tends to last longer than men's and limits activity.
- 42.7 million Americans have osteoarthritis, a painful and debilitating "wear and tear" disease of the joints. Of this number, 26.4 million sufferers are women.
- Of the 10 million people who have fibromyalgia, an arthritis-related syndrome, more than 75 percent are women.
- Women are more likely to experience pain daily than men are (49 percent versus 37 percent, respectively).

Reading the statistics, you might wonder if there is an epidemic of pain in women. There are many reasons for what seems to be an increase in pain reporting by women. First, it could be related to chronic stress, which affects most busy women today who try to juggle families and careers. Alternatively, increased pain could result from biochemical changes in the body from illness, sudden trauma to the central nervous system, or pain-related illnesses such as arthritis or osteoporosis, which are more prevalent in women. Sometimes a deficiency of one of the body's chemicals—serotonin, tryptophan, or even magnesium—may contribute to a lower pain threshold, worsening what would normally be mild or moderate pain.

Still, I contend that there is great hope for women who suffer with chronic pain. The pain can be controlled in most cases, so that you can start to live a normal life again. Of course, ideally you'd like to get rid of the pain by removing the cause or finding a treatment that eliminates it altogether. In many cases, however, that simply cannot be done because cures for many causes of chronic pain, such as fibromyalgia, have not been discovered.

What I *do* know is that most women who have chronic pain *can get relief.* They don't have to simply "live with" the pain anymore, and they can begin to live a normal life again, doing the activities they enjoy. However, the key component in the treatment of chronic pain is *you.* Even if the pain never fully goes away, as soon as you start my 8-step holistic program the chronic pain can become tolerable. In other words, you can change things so that you can get around and do the things you want to do in reasonable comfort, without being severely limited by the pain. You can begin to live your life again, enjoy family and friends, be productive at home and at work—and finally become the master of your pain.

HOWARD SMITH, M.D.

Acknowledgments

In our quest to give accurate and breakthrough information on women and pain, we have received generous contributions from a select group of gifted healthcare professionals, colleagues, family, and friends. We express our gratitude to them all.

Harris H. McIlwain, M.D., rheumatologist and geriatric specialist with Tampa Medical Group, Tampa, Florida, and author of *The Fibromyalgia Handbook* (Holt) and *The Osteoporosis Cure* (Avon): for the latest information on arthritis and osteoporosis.

Jennifer Sippel, R.Ph., pharmacist in Orlando, Florida: for up-to-date information on common medications used to treat pain.

Laura McIlwain-Cruse, M.D.; Kimberly McIlwain, M.D.; Michael F. McIlwain, D.M.D.; Brittnye Bockenek, M.S.; Ashley Elizabeth Bruce; Cristina Yarnoz; Hugh Cruse, M.P.H.; and Sunjay Trehan: for pain research and technical support.

Our agent, Denise Marcil: for enthusiastic support during the inception of this project until the final marketing stage.

Our editor, Elizabeth Zack: for believing in the tremendous need for a compassionate book written for women.

PART I

Taking the Mystery
Out of Women's Pain

CHAPTER ONE

The Women's Pain Epidemic

The latest surveys show that more than 80 million American women suffer each day with some type of chronic pain, such as premenstrual syndrome (PMS) or menstrual pain, back or neck pain, headache, temporomandibular joint syndrome (TMJ), carpal tunnel, and a host of arthritis-related ailments. But no matter what type of pain you have, you know how pain can have an effect on all aspects of life: your marital and family relationships, productivity and ability to earn a living, sleep, eating habits, and overall health. Pain can even stop you from enjoying the little things in life, such as hugging your child or grandchild. When I first spoke to a new patient named Elizabeth at a consultation several years ago, the first thing she said to me was, "Just help me feel good enough to pick up my toddler without hurting all over."

My patient's heartfelt desire may seem unusual to some, but to thirty-six-year-old Elizabeth, who was diagnosed with painful rheumatoid arthritis in her early twenties, having new hope of a pain-free life seemed almost idyllic. Another patient, Janis, also begged for relief of chronic pain. This forty-year-old mother of three is plagued with menstrual migraines that rob her of one week of life each month. "Without fail, two days before my period begins, I wake up with nausea, blurred vision, and the feeling that someone is tightening a relentless steel band around my head. If I don't take my medication immediately, within two hours, I have a full-blown migraine and have to go to bed. I've missed my child's fifth birthday party and a family vacation because of my migraines."

A Woman's Juggling Act

Whether from migraines, menstrual cramps, or childbirth, women experience pain in ways that men cannot even imagine. In fact, in a recent Gallup survey of 2,002 adults over the age of eighteen, researchers reported that 46 percent of women said they had pain daily. In studies presented at the Second International Conference on Women's Health, researchers concluded that women report more pain, more intense pain, and more painful conditions than men do. Researchers also found that women are less likely to receive adequate treatment.

For many women, pain is cyclical. We know that women are much more sensitive than men because of the brain chemistry ebbs and flows, caused by the rise and fall of hormones during the menstrual period. For instance, studies show that women who report more pain during the premenstrual period are more sensitive to pain than women who don't experience PMS.

There are many theories about a woman's greater sensitivity to pain, including speculation that it may be the result of a relative imbalance of serotonin, a naturally occurring neurotransmitter in the body. Serotonin deficiency has been implicated in increased pain, sleep and eating disorders, premenstrual syndrome, menstrual cramps, and depression—all common women's problems. In fact, women experience depression two to three times more often than men do, which researchers believe is related to the lower rate of serotonin synthesis in women. However, the perception of pain is extremely complex and serotonin can also facilitate pain.

Women are also two to three times more likely to have migraine headaches than men are, and these headaches seem to strike whenever estrogen, the neurotransmitter serotonin, and beta-endorphins are low. Likewise, women are six times more likely to have fibromyalgia, an arthritis-related syndrome that results in deep muscle pain and fatigue. More women than men get rheumatoid arthritis, a serious autoimmune disease that results in chronic joint inflammation and pain. In addition, women have the most cases of osteoarthritis, the "wear-and-tear" type of degenerative arthritis that causes chronic pain.

Women Are Undertreated

So, why do doctors seem more willing to treat pain in men than in women? That's a growing concern of women—and their doctors. Some experts believe that women are simply less aggressive than men are in demanding treatment; others believe that many health-care providers regard women as hysterics and feel they overutilize the healthcare system more frequently than men. While this overutilization may have positive results in terms of prevention of disease, some physicians believe the overutilization is obsessive, wasteful, and linked with female "psychological issues." For instance, in one medical center, there were reports of 75 percent of women with endometriosis being dismissed after multiple treatment failures. While all of the women had verified pain, their physicians virtually wrote them off as overutilizers of the healthcare system and dismissed their pain as being "neurotic." In another survey, women with fibromyalgia syndrome (FMS) averaged seeing four to five physicians before receiving a proper diagnosis. Because there are no laboratory tests to show the existence of FMS, the doctors told the women the pain was "in their heads." No matter what anyone tells you, pain is *not* in your head; it is just different in women, and it must be treated effectively for you to reclaim your active life.

The Schulman Study Gives Insight

Perhaps the Schulman study explains why women's pain might be underdiagnosed and treated inadequately. This comprehensive report, published in 1999 in the *New England Journal of Medicine*, studied the relationship of race and gender to physicians' recommendations for managing chest pain. The results of the study were quite revealing and may apply to any medical problem. Study investigators concluded that physicians assessed female patients as being less intelligent, less self-controlled, and more likely to overreport symptoms than male patients. While this bias is *not* intentional, it often results in misdiagnosis and undertreatment for women. In addition, for women with chronic pain, undertreatment sometimes means no life at all.

What Is Pain Anyway?

Pain is an uncomfortable warning sign in your body that lets you know something is wrong. While this feeling is the body's way of alerting the brain that there is a problem, after going on for weeks or months, pain becomes a part of your entire being and existence. At that point, not only is pain a symptom that something is amiss, but pain becomes the disease itself.

How the Brain Perceives Pain

Your body has roughly twenty different nerve endings in the skin that tell you if something is hot, cold, or going to be painful. The nerve endings convey this information to the brain and spinal cord, also known as the central nervous system, to areas where we perceive the stimuli. To accomplish this, the nerve endings of the sensory receptors convert mechanical, thermal, or chemical energy into electrical signals or the painful sensations you actually feel: searing, burning, pounding, or throbbing, among others.

However, pain is more than what you feel at a particular anatomical site. Researchers believe that for women, pain is in your nerves. For instance, in a study in which men and women are subjected to the same irritant, women usually give it a higher pain rating. When pain is chronic or long-term, women usually report insomnia, daytime sleepiness, irritability, appetite loss, muscle weakness, and depression. All of these can make it difficult, if not impossible, to do your daily tasks, including caring for your family and working outside the home. That's why a multifaceted treatment program works well in resolving women's pain instead of relying on a "magic" pill. Moreover, at this writing, there is *no* magic pill.

Chronic or Acute?

It is difficult to think of pain as a positive sign, but it is. Pain is your body's natural signal that there is a potential problem. Without this warning, you might cause irreparable injury. Pain also falls into one of two categories: acute or chronic.

Acute pain comes on suddenly and can be severe. For instance, you know how quickly your back can ache after you've bent down to lift a heavy package or a child. Yet, in more than 80 percent of cases, acute pain goes away in about two weeks; it runs its course and disappears as the problem is relieved. If your pain from a strained muscle lasts only a few days or weeks, it is considered acute.

Chronic pain is acute pain that lasts much longer than would be expected from the original problem or injury. When pain becomes chronic, our bodies react in several ways. Chronic pain may be characterized by brain hormone abnormalities, low energy, mood disorders, muscle pain, and impaired mental and physical performance. The chronic pain worsens as neurochemical changes in the body increase your sensitivity to pain, and you begin to have pain in other parts of the body that do not normally hurt.

Acute pain is important because it brings to our attention a problem that is causing or might cause damage to the body. Acute pain could be a toothache from a cavity in a tooth. It may be a broken bone, a headache from a sinus infection, or a backache from a strain. Muscle pains, joint pain, and pain in the stomach could all be acute signals warning of a potential problem. Some injuries can cause acute pain, such as with bursitis and tendinitis. Each of these types of acute pain "runs its course" and disappears as the problem is relieved.

Surveys have shown that over 70 percent of Americans have acute pain from headaches at some time each year, and over 50 percent have backaches. Acute pain usually lasts a few days to weeks. When the problem is relieved or the injury heals, the pain leaves. For example, acute back pain is so common that most adults in America experience it at some time. In fact, it is the most common cause of loss of work except for the common cold. Acute back pain can come on suddenly and can be severe, but in over 80 percent of cases it goes away in about two to six weeks.

When acute pain lasts for weeks into months, it is called chronic pain, and the body begins to behave differently. Chronic pain prevents sleep, causing you to awaken frequently at night. This results in poor sleep, poor rest, and waking up feeling too tired to start the day. The continued pain causes more irritation and difficulty dealing with others. For women who must take care of family members, work, and cope with chronic pain, life may become too challenging. The overwhelming feelings can lead to irritability, depression, and even suicide for those who feel no hope for relief is in sight.

Pain Is Expensive and Unhealthy

Chronic pain is relentless and expensive, with social costs in disability and lost productivity estimated at more than $100 billion annually. Chronic pain causes nearly 40 million visits to doctors and other health care providers and can extend hospital stays, hinder recovery, and intensely change your quality of life. For women who work outside the home, pain disproportionately affects their productivity and income. While an estimated 36 million Americans missed work in the past year because of pain (27 percent of working adults), women are 50 percent more likely to have missed work because of pain than men are (33 percent versus 22 percent, respectively).

Chronic pain is also unhealthy. Unlike acute pain, which is a sign of a healthy nervous system, chronic pain takes on its own life and mimics a disease. When pain persists for weeks or even months, it can cause an increase in the level of cortisol, the body's main stress-induced hormone. Although a certain amount of cortisol is needed by the immune sysem, when it becomes elevated for an extended period, it can impair the cells that make up your immune system and kidney function.

Because of being bathed in the stress-related chemicals, the immune system can find it harder to function optimally. When you are living with unending chronic pain and the subsequent stress, your immune system simply will not work at full capacity. This breakdown in immune function can interfere with your ability to keep infections at bay, long-term healing, and quality of life. In fact, new studies indicate that pain may cause the growth of cancer cells to speed up when there is pain in the body.

Pain Steals Your Life Away

Then there is the emotional side of a woman's pain. When pain goes on long enough, it can lead to fatigue, insomnia, depression, broken relationships, loss of income, and even suicide. After the removal of a benign brain tumor, fifty-two-year-old Mira was left with what she described as lightninglike pain—and no pain medication could numb it. Because of damage to the trigeminal nerve, one of the main nerves in her face, and the unending pain, Mira never returned to her successful career in computer sales, and she and her husband separated after twenty-two years of marriage. "Without any warning, this burning pain stabs me in the upper jaw and under my eye," Mira said. "I feel as if I'm living with my worst enemy."

LESLIE'S DEEP MUSCLE PAIN AND FATIGUE   When Leslie came for a consultation at my clinic, she was filled with doubt. After seeing seven different doctors over a period of two years about her constant stabbing muscle pain and chronic fatigue, this forty-three-year-old wife and mother was ready to give up any hope of finding relief. "I have real symptoms, but no one can give me a diagnosis," she said. "Doctors have ordered every test imaginable. After the results come in, they shake their heads and say that I'm normal. Dr. Smith, I'm *not* normal!"

After reviewing Leslie's medical records and talking at length with her, I found that she had had a lengthy history of widespread pain for more than two years, experiencing pain in both sides of her body, pain above the waist, and abdominal cramping from time to time. Leslie hurt "everywhere," and she described the pain as "sharp, dull, aching, and pressurelike."

She felt pain when she awoke in the morning, and it seemed to worsen as the day went on. Leslie said just hugging her husband before he left for work brought tears to her eyes because of the muscle pain, and she was in bed resting most evenings so she missed many of her son's soccer games.

After reviewing Leslie's chart and her symptoms, I diagnosed her with fibromyalgia syndrome (FMS)—a group of symptoms that include widespread pain above the waist, below the waist, on the right and left sides of the body, and in the neck or back area. With fibromyalgia, you can have fatigue, insomnia or difficulty maintaining sleep, depression, and a host of other symptoms. There is no cure for fibromyalgia, but you can treat the symptoms with the 8-step program in part 3.

Leslie felt great relief simply by finally getting a diagnosis. Then, once she started the 8-step holistic program, including a low-dose antidepressant to help her improve sleep and a relatively new type of "muscle relaxant" for pain and muscle tightness, this woman reclaimed her active life. She started slowly with exercise, doing stretches for the first week, and then adding brief walks in her neighborhood. She also worked on managing her life better, using a calendar to schedule her days to avoid overextending herself and even opting out of serving on two community committees that "put her in overload." Leslie started eating more healthfully, including more fresh fruits and vegetables and ample protein, and within two months she was a different woman.

The last time Leslie came to the clinic, she was planning a week-long cruise with her husband to celebrate their twentieth wedding anniversary. She realized that with an accurate diagnosis and a multi-faceted treatment plan—including lifestyle changes—she could overcome chronic pain and start to enjoy life again.

ELLEN'S OSTEOARTHRITIS PAIN   At forty-one, Ellen thought she was too young to have arthritis—until she made an appointment to check out severe foot and ankle pain. After college, Ellen was a professional dancer with a large ballet company until she married at age thirty-two. For ten years, she danced almost nightly except for a few brief vacations each year. Little did she know at the time, but the continual pounding on her joints while dancing on a hard stage set her up for early osteoarthritis—the "wear-and-tear" degenerative arthritis that is associated with aging.

Osteoarthritis is more common in adults over fifty, and it affects an estimated 85 percent of the population age seventy and older. Age-related wear and tear and injuries may cause minor damage to the cartilage that will never be completely repaired. The injury might be major and obvious, like a sports-related knee injury, or minor injuries can accumulate over the years and ultimately damage the cartilage, leading to osteoarthritis. Gradually, as more and more damage occurs, the cartilage begins to wear away or doesn't work as well to cushion the joint. As the cartilage cushioning the joint becomes worn, its smoothness is lost, which can cause pain when the joint moves. Along with the pain, you may hear a grating sound when the roughened cartilage on the surface of the bones rubs together.

As for Ellen, she felt the first signs of osteoarthritis in her feet, which began to hurt frequently because osteoarthritis causes the bones to become enlarged. This created added pressure against her shoe and a nearby bone. Other than the pain in her feet and ankles, Ellen felt fine; she had no other pain and had an active lifestyle. After doing blood tests to rule out inflammatory arthritis, I did an X ray of Ellen's ankles and feet, which showed a visible narrowing of the cartilage.

Ellen started the 8-step program in this book and found that with a combination of a Cox-2 inhibitor (Super Aspirin, see page 140), warm water soaks twice daily, and special exercises for her feet, she began to feel better. After two weeks, the pain had diminished. Ellen started walking and swimming for exercise and dropped fifteen pounds, lightening the load for her arthritic feet. This young woman actively involved herself in finding treatment that worked, and she now lives virtually pain-free with only a few reminders of her osteoarthritis when she neglects her daily regimen.

ALLISON'S ABDOMINAL PAIN AND MENSTRUAL CRAMPS   When friends told stories about painful menstrual cramps, Allison knew her personal experience could top any other. At thirty-seven, this young woman had experienced menstrual cramps, along with leg pains, lower back pain, and abdominal cramping for as long as she could remember. In fact, she said she could not recall one menstrual cycle in the past decade when she was pain-free.

After doing a pelvic examination I suspected uterine fibroid tumors, a common tumor that is usually benign. Allison had an ultrasound scan to confirm the diagnosis. Although fibroid tumors are common, they may vary greatly in size. Allison's fibroids were larger than 3 centimeters (bigger than a golf ball) and were the cause of her chronic pelvic pain, painful periods, pelvic pressure, and chronic back pain.

Allison had tried the recommended nonsteroid anti-inflammatory drugs (NSAIDs) to stop the chronic cramping and decrease the blood loss. She then took one of the new Super Aspirins (Cox-2 inhibitors), which are approved for treating menstrual pain. Getting no relief, Allison finally opted for a new procedure called uterine artery embolization to shrink the tumors and end the painful symptoms. This minimally invasive procedure uses techniques similar to those used for a heart catheterization. There are no large incisions, so Allison's recovery only lasted a few days and she was back to work in one week. After the procedure, she rated her menstrual cramping and abdominal pain as very mild and manageable using medication. The best news is that because Allison did not have a hysterectomy to remove the fibroid tumors, she is now pregnant with her first child and thrilled about her new "pain-free" life.

One Size Does Not Fit All

These women's experiences illustrate that women's issues are very different when it comes to the types and intensity of pain, and medications for treating women must be geared appropriately. In the past, doctors used a one-size-fits-all plan to treat pain in women. If you had back pain, you received the same dose of Tylenol 3 as a man.

But is it safe to give a woman who is 5'2" and weighs 110 pounds the same dose as a 6'4", 220-pound male? Some experts are now saying no. Additionally, even when women and men are the same size, it appears that various medications work somewhat differently in females than in males. Studies are finally underway to find the proper dosages for women. Also, women may respond differently than men to medications. It seems that potent narcotics that strongly stimulate the kappa narcotic receptor may work better in general for women's pain than potent narcotics that strongly stimulate the mu narcotic receptor.

For women who wonder why over-the-counter nonsteroid anti-inflammatory drugs (NSAIDs), such as Advil, don't always work to relieve pain, there is a reason. Some new findings indicate that NSAIDs might be ineffective for pain during the first two weeks of a woman's menstrual cycle. (Ironically, this finding is not shown on the ibuprofen packaging!) Because chronic pain is different for women, and women are *not* just small men, this field demands specialized understanding, prevention, treatment, and medication—all given to you in the 8-step program in this book.

A Multifaceted Program Is the Key

Unlike other books on the subject of pain, this book places *you* at center stage by focusing on how to relieve pain common in women. The steps to ending this pain need not be intrusive or include powerful, mind-altering drugs that can reduce energy and alertness. Instead, I know that a multifaceted holistic program is the only way to help many women end chronic pain. As you read this book, you will see that it quickly moves beyond the descriptions of common types of pain and on to pages of self-help tips that you can use today to feel better. The program I recommend to my patients will give you the most effective medical, low-tech, high-tech, natural, and alternative approaches to stopping pain and reversing painful symptoms without side effects—for women.

When writing this book, we had three major goals:

1. To educate women on how the unique effect of hormones on a woman's nervous system can influence pain and how pain can affect every part of her being—physical, mental, emotional, and spiritual. Therefore, I believe that a woman's pain mandates a

scientifically sound but holistic treatment plan that helps her heal in all these areas.

2. To help women identify the specific type of pain they have, whether backache, headache, menstrual pain, fibromyalgia, osteoarthritis, osteoporosis, or everyday aches and pains, and understand why they feel this pain differently than their male counterparts.

3. To provide an 8-step holistic program to stop pain and reverse painful symptoms by guiding women through a crucial diagnostic process and toward finding the most effective medications, natural therapies, dietary treatments, mind/body therapies, and high-tech gadgets or surgical interventions, if needed.

I believe I've accomplished those goals and more in the 8-step program, and I know the numerous therapies will help you. From years of academic studies and clinical experience, I have found that often "less is more" when it comes to treating pain. In that regard, I sometimes take an unconventional path to help women get relief without the intruding side effects of strong pain medications. For instance, I may suggest a "cocktail" of ground pain relievers blended in a cream base (these can be made in a compounding pharmacy; more on this later). This substance helps the pain relievers to get through the skin, directly to the painful site. Because the medication is topical (on the skin) and not directly systemic (in the bloodstream), you can get relief without the drowsiness of normal pain medications. After all, who can afford to be drowsy when you are balancing career, family, and other commitments?

In this book, I will teach you how lifestyle habits and self-care can increase or decrease pain, and how making a few small changes in habits can give tremendous pain-relieving results. For example, studies show that deep stage-4 sleep can alleviate the pain you feel, while an increase in life's stressors can super-charge your body's pain response, making the pain you feel worse than normal. For reasons unknown, studies find that inactive or sedentary women have more pain while physically active women have fewer pain disorders. That's why it takes a combination of conventional medical treatments and alternative lifestyle strategies to help you get back in control of your sleep, stress, physical activity, and more. I want you to reclaim your active life—without any pain.

I'll also help you to get focused so that when you visit your doctor, you can relay clearly what you are experiencing and get optimal treatment. If you aren't happy with your doctor's response, *call another doctor.* Seek another opinion until you find the best relief of pain and other symptoms.

Now before I discuss the many common types of pain women feel and the treatments to resolve these, let's look at the cycle of pain in chapter 2, which discusses how pain can wreak havoc with your emotional state—until you get back in control.

CHAPTER TWO

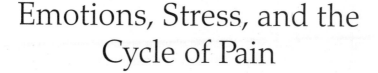

Emotions, Stress, and the Cycle of Pain

Where do you go when it hurts? If you're like many women with pain, there's really no place to hide. Annie, a forty-three-year-old magazine editor, said she suffered for months with relentless carpal tunnel syndrome (CTS). In this condition the median nerve, which travels down the arm into the hand, becomes compressed as it passes through the bones and connective tissue in the wrist that form the "carpal tunnel." Overuse causes the tissues in the area to swell, and this swelling causes added pressure on the median nerve.

Annie took nonsteroid anti-inflammatory drugs (NSAIDs) to decrease inflammation and pain and used moist heat wraps as recommended. She also wore a wrist splint at night. Still, without fail, she woke up during the night with pain, tingling, and numbness in her thumb and fingers. Sometimes the pain traveled up her arm to her elbow, making it impossible for her to rest comfortably.

While Annie was following "the doctor's orders" for treating her CTS, I told her that unless she stopped the daytime abuse of her wrist, she might have to face a surgical procedure. She knew having surgery meant taking time off from her job and having to stop using the wrist for several weeks. I reminded Annie that if she used the wrist pad on her computer keyboard and let her children help carry in heavy packages and do any household chores that might cause repetitive strain on her wrist, the carpal tunnel syndrome would probably heal and the pain would resolve.

Annie thought it was virtually impossible to stop using her wrist, especially since her kids were young and still depended on her. Nevertheless, she made it a point to tape her wrist or wear her wrist splint in the daytime hours as a reminder to avoid overuse. She told her children that when they saw the wrist splint, they were to watch their mom cautiously to make sure she did not overuse her wrist. Annie's husband started helping with the dishes and heavy chores. Within a month of letting the wrist rest, Annie told me the pain and numbness had stopped.

Women Ignore Self-Care

I know how difficult it is to stop all your responsibilities to others and take care of yourself. Because of your special biological makeup, women are the caregivers and nurturers of family and friends. Newly published research suggests that the neurohormone oxytocin, which plays a key role in the initiation of maternal behavior in conjunction with female reproductive hormones, may be at the core of a woman's "tend and befriend" nurturing pattern. In other words, this response may not be something you can change without some definite effort. In my clinical experience, I've seen how many women, even those with the most intense pain, tend to put caring for themselves on the back burner. Yet, as they focus on caring for the immediate needs of family and friends, along with their overly extended list of commitments, they cheat themselves out of resolving the pain and enjoying an active life.

How can a young mother who suffers with chronic migraines get relief when she spends her days chasing a toddler and carpooling older children to school and extracurricular activities? How can a single, middle-aged woman with back and neck pain from osteoarthritis follow her doctor's advice if she works full time to earn a living, and cares for her aging parents when she gets home? In addition, consider the woman who suffers with severe menstrual cramps for days each month, yet teaches school fulltime and then goes home to cook and clean for her large family. How does she get resolution of her debilitating and regular monthly pain?

Pain Is an Intrapersonal Experience

One of the first questions many women who come to the clinic ask is, "Doctor, am I overreacting to the pain?"

Sometimes well-meaning friends or family members mention in jest that the pain is "all in your head." In fact, you may have heard the following statements:

"You look fine! Just think pleasant thoughts and maybe you won't think about your pain."

"I can't imagine pain lasting this long. Are you sure your doctor didn't misdiagnose you?"

"Just put the pain out of your mind, and get busy with some project. You'll forget about it soon."

"Maybe if you exercised (lost weight, got more rest), your pain would subside."

"Aren't you being a bit overreactive? I mean, you always had a big imagination as a child."

"Maybe that new medicine the doctor gave you is worsening the pain. Why don't you try going without any medicine?"

After living so long with pain, you may start to wonder if you really *are* imagining it! Or perhaps you left your doctor's office with hope that the newly prescribed medication would do the trick this time and stop your pain. Then when the pain was worse than ever several days later, you began to wonder if the pain wasn't really in your head, as one friend had suggested. Or, maybe your pain stopped for a few days or weeks, and you just knew you were healed. Then, when the pain started again, you felt like giving up and wondered what you had done wrong to deserve this.

No matter what friends or family members tell you, you must know that the pain is not in your head; it is very real. In chapter 1, I discussed the feelings of pain and how pain is undertreated in women, even though women often experience more pain than men do. It's important also to understand that chronic pain is an intrapersonal experience, not just a diagnosis. This means chronic pain encompasses everything about you—your feelings, emotions, attitude, as well as the actual pain you feel. Once you understand the various emotions that coincide with your pain problem, you can set goals to move beyond your negative feelings by developing an optimistic, resilient attitude as you undertake the 8-step holistic program.

The Emotions of Chronic Pain

If your pain has lasted for months, you may have forgotten what it was like to be happy, carefree, and optimistic—even though you were a positive person before your pain began. Diane's story is typical of most women with chronic pain. This forty-three-year-old single mother suffered with menstrual migraines for more than seven years until a combination of medication, eliminating trigger foods, and biofeedback helped her gain control.

I was in my mid-thirties when the chronic migraines started. I had never had a bad headache, at least one that aspirin didn't resolve. The pain was frightening. I remember it coming on suddenly, and it felt like electricity shooting through my eyes—so much that I had to close my eyes and lie still with a cold cloth on my head for hours until I was able to function.

Hoping the headache was acute, I talked to my doctor who recommended nonsteroid anti-inflammatory drugs to help decrease inflammation and pain. Therefore, when the second migraine happened—about one month later—I took Advil, which did nothing to stop the pain. I saw three doctors and tried every medication they suggested over a seven-year period. I just knew there'd be an end to my suffering; after all, I was healthy, resilient, and had excellent coping skills.

Then each month, as the menstrual migraine came back, the constant pain—or anticipation of pain—wore me down. My coping skills weakened, and I started to live in an emotional world filled with anxiety, fear, depression, and other problems. The pain literally controlled me, and I took my negative emotions out on my son and coworkers.

Then there is Laura, a thirty-three-year-old mother of three, who suffered for years with chronic neck and back pain. Because the pain medications her doctor gave her made her dizzy and drowsy, she tried not to take them unless she was desperate for relief. Without the right medications, Laura's pain was undertreated, and it began to invade every part of her life—from her sleep to her daily activities to her diet to her mood. After her third child was born, Laura was determined to find an answer to her pain problem and sought help from alternative medicine practitioners, hoping for a natural cure. The cost of these appointments and the time they took, combined with the episodes of severe pain and poor sleep, added to Laura's physical and emotional distress.

Almost a year passed, and Laura started taking narcotic pain medications without her doctor's supervision. The drugs made her want to sleep and she spent more time in bed, hiring the teenager next door to watch her children in the afternoon so she could rest. When Laura hurt so badly that she could not stand without severe back pain, her husband took a leave from his job to stay home with the children. The stress of the loss of income, along with Laura's illness and narcotic addiction, caused relationship problems. Laura and her husband divorced after a few months. He now keeps the children at his apartment, because she is unable to be a healthy parent.

I don't deny that emotional stress can trigger a host of health-related problems, ranging from memory loss to impaired immunity. It definitely plays a role in pain-related problems. Chronic pain *is* emotional—it affects every part of your being. However, there are easy steps you can take to counter these emotions. So let's start by discussing common factors associated with chronic pain that can result in negative emotions. Once you understand these factors, you can then focus on positive ways to release the destructive emotions and move forward toward health and healing.

Anxiety and Fear

Most women with pain live in a constant state of anxiety and fear. Not only is the pain frightening when it intensifies for no reason, but the fear of the unknown can be overwhelming.

When you become obsessive about your fears and focus on what "might happen," you become an obstacle in your quest to conquer the pain. High anxiety can lead to poor sleep, which can result in more pain the next day. Dwelling on fears can lead to feelings of sadness and make you want to be alone, as you stay isolated from family and friends.

You may lie awake at night, wondering if your pain will worsen and how you will handle that. You may also worry that your pain is caused by a more serious problem that your doctor has not yet diagnosed. On the other hand, you might be afraid that you'll have to quit your job because of the constant pain or have to find help to raise your children. Some women worry that their husbands or significant others will abandon them and seek a relationship with a healthy woman.

Anger

After suffering for months to years with unresolved pain, many women harbor unresolved anger. I explain to patients that anger is a normal reaction to any chronic or long-term health problem, but how we respond to anger can vary.

Just as holding anger inside or "stuffing" your feelings is unhealthy, so is letting angry feelings consume your entire being. Some women who stifle their anger hold their deepest emotions inside, then lash out at unsuspecting family members or friends. Others are outwardly anger and bitter because of their "plight" in life, which seems so unfair. Some women blame their physicians for not having the proper treatment to resolve their pain, even though no such treatment exists.

Social Isolation

Granted, you may intentionally avoid some people because you simply don't feel good. But spending too much time alone can be an indication of a greater problem—social isolation.

I know you're tired, irritable, and more than anything else, you hurt. On the one hand, you may be purposely avoiding some people or the problems you have in order to face each day. In that case, it's easy to find your home a secure haven where you are not on display and where there are loved ones around to meet your needs. On the other hand, loss of desire to be with friends and decreased social support are common warning signs of depression. In that case, you may want to consider professional help.

There's always the chance that some friends may be avoiding you, especially if you are constantly updating them on your pain and health situation. I'm sure your friends care deeply for you and want to know how you feel, but if all you talk about is your physical health, you may find the telephone ringing less and less often as time passes.

Stress

Stress describes the many demands and pressures that all people experience to some degree each day. These demands may be physical, mental, emotional, or even chemical in nature. We use the word "stress" to include both the stressful situation known as the "stressor" and the symptoms you experience under stress that are your "stress response."

Physical discomfort resulting from psychosocial stress is one of the most common reasons why people seek medical care. A revealing twenty-year study at Kaiser Permanente concluded that more than

60 percent of their medical visits were by the "worried well," with no diagnosable medical condition. Not surprisingly, the United States Public Health Service estimates that 70 percent of the current health-care budget is spent treating individuals with chronic diseases—many caused by negative lifestyle habits or chronic stress.

Just about anything you encounter can cause stress. I've found with most patients that it's not life's emergencies or disasters that trigger the majority of stress reactions, but the persistent interruptions, hassles, and struggles of everyday living. Whether you are confronted with financial problems, waiting in long lines of traffic each evening, or raising active children, all can add up to be overwhelming stress, triggering additional pain.

When your stress and pain escalate over time, they can create even further problems, including:

- Difficulty sleeping, leading to constant fatigue
- Inability to exercise, leading to poor aerobic and physical fitness
- Difficulty concentrating from the side effects of medications, leading to poor performance
- Increased irritability from lack of sleep or medications' side-effects
- Withdrawal from favorite activities because of low energy
- Changes in appetite due to medications
- Depression

The fact is, stress is simply the trigger. Your response to stress is what influences your pain level, as well as other aspects of your physical and emotional health. For example, when emotional stress overwhelms you, your immune system, heart and blood vessels, and certain glands secrete hormones that help regulate various functions in the body, such as brain function and nerve impulses. All of these responses interact and are strongly influenced by your coping skills and mental state. Yet, if you react inappropriately to the stressor, the pain you feel can be intensified.

"Stress is nothing new to me," you might say. "I live with it daily and have suffered its consequences." Yes, stress is here to stay. However, no two people respond in the same way to all stressful events. People perceive and respond to stressors in different ways, and inappropriate responses may influence your health.

Stress activates the sympathetic nervous system, stimulating the release of hormones such as cortisol. A constant saturation of this results in many physiologic changes that help you fight or flee in an emergency. Yet these changes—including increased heart rate, breathing, and blood pressure—can tear down your body's immune system and ability to ward off illness. Under normal conditions these changes subside quickly, but chronic stressors, including anxiety, fear, anger, and grief, can keep the nervous system perpetually aroused. Prolonged stress has been found to contribute to illness and immune changes in both human and animal models.

Given the evidence that stress increases the pain you feel, it seems logical to presume that decreasing stress can modulate pain. We all know that when we have peaceful thoughts, we tend to have a comparable emotional reaction and similar physiological reaction as well; we feel in control of our life and our health. When we have angry or anxious thoughts, we tend to be emotionally aroused. Consequently, our physiological reactions are more dramatic, and we are prone to making bad health choices such as eating foods that are not healthful, smoking cigarettes, or abusing alcohol or drugs. An increasing number of physicians, psychiatrists, and psychologists are acknowledging that the way we think, feel, act, and react can be a powerful determinant of our physical and mental health.

For those with chronic pain, the negative stress cycle can be difficult to interrupt, so it's better not to get caught up in the first place. Your stress response may be chronic back or neck pain. On the other hand, maybe you suffer with migraines or tension headaches when life's stressors become overwhelming. Whatever your stress response, learn to identify your stress warning signals, which are cues to the start of symptoms. By paying attention to these signals, you can recognize when the chronic pain cycle is about to begin and adopt effective prevention strategies.

FIVE SIGNS YOUR STRESS LEVEL IS HIGH

1. You are irritable and edgy.
2. Your sleep habits change; you sleep too much or you cannot sleep at all.
3. You don't feel happy. Your feeling of fulfillment or joy is gone.
4. Your eating habits change; you eat too much or you cannot eat at all.

5. You have relationship problems at home, with friends, and at work.

Check the stress symptoms you experience when under stress. These are your personal stress warning signals. Once you can recognize these, you can take steps to reduce your stress, using the steps in the 8-step program.

STRESS SYMPTOM ASSESSMENT

_____ 1. I feel tired or run down.

_____ 2. I get angry or frustrated easily.

_____ 3. I cannot concentrate at work.

_____ 4. Little things agitate me, and I feel like screaming.

_____ 5. I get headaches or stomachaches regularly.

_____ 6. I awaken frequently at night, thinking about my problems.

_____ 7. I feel sad or unhappy frequently.

_____ 8. I don't have a sense of humor and rarely laugh.

_____ 9. I am highly critical of everyone around me.

_____ 10. I feel overwhelmed.

_____ 11. I frequently use alcohol to soothe my nerves.

_____ 12. I clench my jaws while sleeping.

_____ 13. I have lost or gained more than ten pounds recently.

_____ 14. I feel hopeless.

_____ 15. I'm very disorganized and cannot remember where I put things.

Seeking Social Support

While there is no quick fix for resolving any of the detrimental emotions of chronic pain, you can take measures to deal with these in a positive way, so they do not hinder your personal goals and relationships. In this book, I give you countless ways to reduce stress, including physical exercise, mind/body modalities, and massage and other touch therapies. However, I also want you to consider the healing impact of social support. There are new findings that social support is important for those with chronic illnesses. I believe the same is true for women with chronic pain. Social support may be defined as the sum of all the relationships that make you feel as if you matter to the people who matter to you. Studies have verified that a strong group of family members and close friends or a support system (doctors, nurses, other health care professionals) can help in coping with a chronic illness. In some cases, having this social strength has been associated with people's greater adherence to medical regimens and use of health services.

You know how stress supercharges you, causing stomach distress and aches and pains, or sending your heart rate soaring. In the same way, social support has a complex effect on well-being—but it is calming and positive. Social support may change your assessment of the stressful event or may prevent you from engaging in damaging behavioral or physiological responses.

How Does It Work?

When you are tied emotionally to those in your social network, you can express your feelings of fear, insecurity, and guilt and receive comfort from people who accept you just as you are, with no strings attached. If you have no place that feels safe enough to let down your emotional defenses, you tend to keep your guard up all the time—a negative, cynical, and sometimes defensive guard that masks the very problems you are facing.

With increased social support, you can alleviate the emotional distress of chronic pain and gain health benefits, such as the following:

- *Sense of control.*   While you may have no control over your chronic pain, having a group of supportive family members and friends is something you can control.

- *Greater resilience.*   Through positive feedback and support from friends and family, you learn to buffer life's interruptions with effective coping skills instead of letting the moment's crisis overwhelm you.

- *Longevity.*   In study after study, the findings are the same: people with many social contacts—a spouse or partner, a close-knit family, a network of friends, religious or other group affiliations—lived longer and had better health. Those who had few ties with other people died at rates two to five times higher than those with good social ties.

Evaluate Your Social Network

I'd like you to look at your social network and make sure you have comfortable support in the following key areas: emotional, social, informational, and practical.

1. *Emotional support.* Do you have a friend who is a confidant and who you can trust with your most personal feelings and worries?
2. *Social support.* Do you have a friend you enjoy being with, who helps you survive disappointments and who understands your pain?
3. *Informational support.* Do you have someone you can ask for advice on major decisions?
4. *Practical support.* Do you have a friend who will help you out in a pinch?

I'll give you more information on seeking social support in Step 8, when I discuss the importance of support groups. For now, just make sure your social network is strong and that you have close friends you can lean on in times of distress.

Now Rate Your Pain

Before I discuss the most common types of pain women experience, I want to help you rate the pain you feel. This is important, as your doctor will want to know how you feel and if you can describe your pain and how it affects your life, you'll be able to respond to treatment more rapidly.

When I ask my patients to tell me about their pain, almost all of them instantly reply, "It hurts!" Of course, it hurts. Pain is painful! I find it helpful for patients to rate their pain so they can measure their own progress as they embark on the 8-step program. I devised the following Smith Pain Quotient (SPQ). Using this scale, you can keep a month-long calendar and rate your pain on a daily basis to see if it is improving or worsening. If you are following the 8-step program, along with your doctor's prescribed medications, and your pain has increased, call your doctor for an evaluation. You may need a change of medication, or there may be another reason for the pain.

SMITH PAIN QUOTIENT (SPQ)

To find your SPQ, start by circling a number that reflects how much pain you feel today.

0 = no pain ◄———► 10 = worst pain imaginable

0   1   2   3   4   5   6   7   8   9   10

Now circle a number that reflects how the pain you feel interferes with each of the nine following areas:

Ability to walk

0   1   2   3   4   5   6   7   8   9   10

Activities of daily living

0   1   2   3   4   5   6   7   8   9   10

Mood

0   1   2   3   4   5   6   7   8   9   10

Sleep

0   1   2   3   4   5   6   7   8   9   10

Enjoyment of life

0   1   2   3   4   5   6   7   8   9   10

Relationship with significant other(s)

0   1   2   3   4   5   6   7   8   9   10

Recreational activities

0   1   2   3   4   5   6   7   8   9   10

Sexual activities

0   1   2   3   4   5   6   7   8   9   10

Amount of social interaction

0   1   2   3   4   5   6   7   8   9   10

Calculate Your SPQ

Now add together all the numbers you circled and divide by ten. The resulting quotient is your Smith Pain Quotient (SPQ). Calculate your SPQ daily for a week, and keep track of this number. Then, start my 8-

step holistic program, and continue to calculate your SPQ weekly as you progress. If your score decreases, that's a sign that you are showing improvement and starting to enjoy facets of your life again. If the score increases or you become dissatisfied with the program, check with your doctor for additional advice.

Knowledge Is Crucial

When I consult with women in pain, much of their anxiety and fears stem from a lack of knowledge about chronic pain and their particular disease or problem. Not only are they hurting, but the distress of living with a chronic ailment is frightening. Misconceptions keep many women from taking action when pain becomes overwhelming, and they fear a diagnosis. Education helps them to move beyond these fears.

In the next six chapters, I discuss some of the most common types of pain in women. Within each chapter, I detail what causes the pain, what symptoms you might feel, how it's diagnosed, and how the pain is treated. Use these chapters to further your understanding of your pain and the specific remedies for treating the pain. Then carefully review my 8-step holistic program for the ins-and-outs of how the specific pain problem, is diagnosed and treated, and the therapies that might work best for you. Then make an appointment with your doctor to talk about your signs and symptoms, as well as the myriad medications or high-tech procedures that are discussed. You will realize that a multifaceted approach to resolving or managing chronic pain is the best form of treatment, as it lets you become the master of your pain—and of your life.

Now let's get started!

PART II

Identifying Your Pain

CHAPTER THREE

Back and Neck Pain

"Doctor, my back is killing me" is a common complaint. Younger women experience back pain frequently with premenstrual syndrome, menstrual cramping and aches, or from the strain of lifting young children. Middle-aged and older women often have back pain from injuries, disc disease, or degenerative diseases such as arthritis or osteoporosis.

Many women also suffer needlessly with neck pain, whether from a past injury, poor posture, computer strain, or fibromyalgia (an arthritis-related syndrome that causes deep muscle pain). Like back pain, neck pain can also stem from osteoporosis, arthritis, and disc diseases.

MEREDITH BECAME THE MASTER OF HER PAIN   Meredith, a forty-three-year-old teacher and mother of two, was playing in an amateur tennis tournament when she experienced excruciating back pain as she twisted her body while using her new backhand swing. Initially the pain was sharp and penetrating, pulsating down her right leg like an electric shock—severe enough to make Meredith forfeit her game. Within hours of the injury, Meredith's entire right leg and foot were numb, and she was unable to sleep that night due to the severity of pain, which now ascended to the back of her neck and shoulders. The pain worsened when she sat or bent forward and lessened when she reclined.

When Meredith came to see me the following morning, I ordered a test called magnetic resonance imaging (MRI), a special imaging technique used to image internal structures of the body. It showed a ruptured disc in her lower lumbar spine. Agreeing to use self-care methods to get fast relief, Meredith began using regular compresses of ice on her lower back and neck, along with anti-inflammatory medications (NSAIDs) to help alleviate the inflammation and reduce the pain. She then started easy stretching exercises (as explained in Step 4) and began a walking program of fifteen minutes each day. Within two weeks, she was able to do most of her usual routine at home and at school. Moreover, after three weeks of self-care, Meredith showed great improvement and increased her exercise and activity. (For women who continue with severe pain despite conservative measures, an injection of corticosteroids into the epidural space in the back may be helpful, as discussed in Step 8.)

If you suffer with neck or back pain (or both), it's important to become the master of your pain by seeking an accurate diagnosis, and then using healing therapies. Let's look further at both types of pain and the recommended remedies to resolve them.

Back Pain

When I first saw Jessica, she had been suffering with lower back pain in the lumbar spine for more than four years, since her last pregnancy. Yet Jessica's pain was tricky. This thirty-eight-year-old mother of two described how the lower back pain sometimes affected the middle and upper parts of the back. Other times the pain would radiate down her legs to the feet, feeling almost like electricity. Sometimes she had pain in her hip or numbness in her feet and toes because of the referred pain.

What You Might Feel: Signs and Symptoms

Jessica's symptoms were typical of back pain. No matter what type of back pain you have, you may feel typical or atypical symptoms, including the following:

- Severe pain (sharp, shooting, or the electric-shock type) in the back
- Pain that is felt in the lower back and down the back of one leg
- Numbness or tingling
- Inability to point or extend big toe on the foot that has leg pain

- Weakness of certain leg or foot muscles
- Disturbance of the normal heel-toe gait, that is, inability to walk on one foot or foot-drop (a foot that essentially "drags" along due to dysfunction of the muscles which normally "pull" your foot/toes up toward your head)
- Severe pain (sharp, shooting, or the electrical-shock type) in back of neck, shoulder, or down one arm
- Pain that worsens with movement or activity
- Numbness or tingling in one arm
- Weakness of arm muscles

What Causes Back Pain?

Computer Users Are at High Risk.   There are many common causes of back pain in women, such as muscle aches, muscle strain, poor posture, menstrual cramps, premenstrual syndrome, and bladder infections, among others. Did you know that more than half of all computer users report some type of neck or back pain each year? Researchers from Emory University studied men and women who used computers more than fifteen hours a week over a three-year period. Their findings, published in the *American Journal of Industrial Medicine*, stated that more women than men reported an injury or problem, and one-third of computer users actually developed an impairment or loss of function.

Disc Disease Is a Common Cause.   Disc disease is another common cause of back pain. Discs are the small cushions that separate the bony spinal vertebrae. You might think of your discs as small shock absorbers for the spine. When a disc ruptures, there is a gradual or sudden break in the supportive ligaments surrounding it. Common causes include sustaining a sudden injury (when you lift too much weight) or constant stress (obesity). When a disc ruptures, the disc material can cause pressure or irritation to one of the sciatic nerves, a pair of nerves that pass through the pelvis and travel down the back of each thigh. That is why a ruptured disc can hurt all the way down to your feet.

If you like to do stretches in the morning, you may want to wait a few hours if you suffer with back pain. There appears to be a greater risk of insult to the structures of the spine and lower back with significant bending forward in the early morning. Wait until you've warmed up, and then slowly begin your exercise routine to avoid further injury.

Sometimes the Cause Is Unknown.   Sometimes the pain may be called "acute lower back (lumbar) strain," but the cause may be from an injury or may not be apparent at all. At times there may be pressure on a nerve in the lower back. Some internal organ problems can make pain travel to the back and are disguised as back pain. An atypical sign of heart attack in women is upper back pain. In addition, such problems as peptic ulcer disease (stomach ulcer), pancreatitis, and gallstones can cause back pain.

Osteoarthritis is another common cause of back pain, especially in women over age forty. Osteoporosis (thinning of the bones), discussed in chapter 9, may also cause severe back pain when a bone fractures in the back. Other serious problems that can cause back pain include enlargement of the aorta (aortic aneurysm), some forms of cancer, and kidney problems. Each of these needs proper diagnosis and treatment. The best idea is to check with your doctor to be sure no other causes of back pain are present.

Other reasons your back may hurt include the following:

- Incorrect lifting
- An accident, recreational sports injury, or sudden fall
- Poor muscle tone
- Excessive body weight, particularly a protruding stomach
- Sitting in one position for a long time
- Carrying a heavy purse or shoulder bag
- Chronic stress

Sometimes back problems stem from instability or dysfunction of various anatomical structures, including:

- Zygapophyseal (facet) joints. The zygapophyseal joints are the spine joints (one on the right side and one on the left side) which join the lower portions of a vertebral body above with the upper portions of a vertebral body below—throughout the spine. This pain is often felt across the very low back, radiating to the upper back of the thigh. Usually bending backwards aggravates this condition, and bending forward helps.
- Spinal stenosis. This is a narrowing of the spine most often seen in the elderly, giving rise to pain mostly with walking. With rest, the pain generally subsides. Learning forward slightly as when pushing a shopping cart seems to help.
- Sacroiliac joints. This pain is felt over the sacroiliac region in the lower back, hips, or groin.

- Internal disc disruption or problems. "Discogenic" pain makes sitting almost intolerable; standing can make it feel better.

RISK FACTORS FOR RUPTURED OR HERNIATED DISC

- Participating in a sport or recreational activity (bowling, tennis, running, jogging, football, soccer, racquetball, weight-lifting, gymnastics) that causes a downward pressure on the neck or spine
- Being in poor physical condition
- Warming up improperly before exercise or activity
- Being obese
- Having a family history of back pain or disc disorders
- Lifting heavy items and using poor lifting techniques

How Back Pain Is Diagnosed

I diagnose the cause of back pain after much discussion with the patient and after a full physical examination and specific tests. Starting with a detailed medical history, I find out about the patient's symptoms, including how she feels, her activity level, her diet, her home and work environment, and her medical and family history. The medical examination usually includes a physical exam, lab test, and X rays or scans, as explained in Step 1. I encourage the patient to openly talk with me about her symptoms and concerns, providing all the details about the condition that will contribute to an accurate diagnosis such as any recent falls. I then order the appropriate test to confirm the diagnosis. Commonly used tests to diagnose back pain include X rays, myelography, magnetic resonance imaging (MRI), computed tomography (CT) scan, bone scan, and electrodiagnostic studies.

Neck Pain

Whether from osteoarthritis, degenerative disc disease, an injury, or constant straining while sitting at a computer terminal all day, neck pain can interfere with your activities and daily routine. In most cases, neck pain is acute and resolves in a few days or weeks. Yet for those women who have chronic neck pain, the pain can be excruciating and may limit quality of life, including sleep and exercise.

What You Might Feel: Signs and Symptoms

You may feel dull or sharp pain in the neck. It may be stabbing, piercing, cramping, or burning. At first the neck pain may be mild. Then, over the course of a few hours or days, the pain may worsen. You may also have muscle weakness, numbness, or swelling in the neck along with the pain.

What Causes Neck Pain?

Neck pain happens when you sprain the muscles, tendons, and ligaments of your neck or shoulders. This may be the result of an accident or injury to the neck muscles and ligaments. In some cases, the spinal cord, heart, lungs, and some abdominal organs also can cause neck and shoulder pain. Poor posture may also result in neck pain, as can muscle tension from chronic stress. When there is a known specific injury, the neck pain and stiffness usually occurs within days of the event.

With a severe injury, the more likely there is damage to the muscles, tendons, and ligaments in the neck. For instance, a whiplash injury to the neck from an automobile accident throws the head backward or forward, followed by a sudden rebound movement in the opposite direction.

The stronger the force on the neck, the more injury there is to the "soft tissues" and the more severe your pain may be. The injury may lead to problems with the cervical zygapophyseal (facet) joints, which seems to be the source of pain for a majority of whiplash injuries.

Other areas in the neck and head can have injury, including injury to the jaw (temporomandibular) joint or other structures, dislocations of joints, or small fractures in the bones of the spine. In severe injuries, there may be damage to the nerves in the neck or the spinal cord.

Trigger points, localized areas around muscles and other tissue in the neck that are painful when pressure is applied, may cause pain that travels down one arm and can mimic pressure on a nerve in the neck. If left untreated, these trigger areas may be very long-lasting and a major cause of chronic neck pain.

Arthritis can cause pain and stiffness in joints and may also affect the neck. The most common type is osteoarthritis (discussed in chapter 8). Osteoarthritis causes the discs and cartilage of the joints between the bones in the neck to become thin and worn, resulting in pain and stiffness. Sometimes bony outgrowths called "spurs" can form, making it painful to move your neck. After changing your head and neck positioning to compensate for the arthritis pain, you may develop even more strain and achiness.

Rheumatoid arthritis is another cause of neck pain. This more serious inflammatory arthritis can attack the neck, where it causes pain, stiffness and headaches and makes it difficult to turn the neck. In severe cases, the spine may become so damaged that surgery is needed.

Long-term wear and tear may result in pressure on a nerve that travels down one or both arms and sometimes even the fingers. Along with the neck pain, you may have a feeling of numbness or tingling that travels down your arm. The feeling may be like pins and needles in the arms or feel as if the arm has "fallen asleep."

The most common cause of pressure on a nerve as it leaves the spinal cord is a ruptured disc in the neck, cervical osteoarthritis, or injury. This can cause severe neck pain that may be disabling.

How Is Neck Pain Diagnosed?

Your doctor will take a medical history, including details of how you injured your neck or when it started hurting. Tests, which may include X rays, magnetic resonance imaging, and CT scan are helpful in making the diagnosis, especially in finding if there is pressure on a nerve in the neck. Other tests such as electromyography (EMG) and myelography are sometimes used if nerve damage is suspected.

Treating Back and Neck Pain

Medications

Because many causes of back or neck pain stem from inflammation, you may find that a nonsteroidal anti-inflammatory drug (NSAID) gives immediate relief and reduces this inflammation. Some common anti-inflammatory medications are ibuprofen (Advil, Motrin), flurbiprofen (Ansaid), nabumetone (Relafen), and etodolac (Lodine). The new Super Aspirins (Cox-2 inhibitors), such as valdecoxib (Bextra), rofecoxib (Vioxx), and celecoxib (Celebrex) may give excellent relief from pain, too. These prescription medications are less likely to upset the stomach than other NSAIDs.

Sometimes I prescribe antidepressants for back or neck pain because they also have a pain-relieving effect and can help improve sleep and speed recovery. Muscle relaxants, such as cyclobenzaprine hydrochloride (Flexeril), orphenadrine citrate (Norflex), metaxalone (Skelaxin), carisoprodol (Soma) and diazepam (Valium), are prescription medications that may help if you are having muscle spasms in the neck or back. While these medications may help you sleep more soundly, they may not give relief from pain unless you have a spasm. Longer-term medications may include tizanidine hydrochloride (Zanaflex) and baclofen (Lioresal).

Various medications available for controlling relentless back or neck pain require a prescription from your doctor. These include narcotics such as propoxyphene hydrochloride (Darvon), propoxyphene with acetaminophen (Darvocet), codeine with acetaminophen (Phenaphen #3 or Tylenol #3) and hydrocodone with acetaminophen (Lortab, Vicodin), among others. Because narcotic pain medications may lead to dependency issues, your doctor may limit these to short-term use for severe pain only. You may then be given an analgesic, such as acetaminophen, or a nonsteroid anti-inflammatory.

Some prescription medications are nonnarcotic, so they are less likely to be habit forming, such as ketorolac tromethamine (Toradol), which is available by injection or tablet. This medication is intended for short-term use for pain control. Another prescription tablet for pain control is tramadol hydrochloride (Ultram). Over-the-counter (no prescription needed) analgesics or pain relievers, including acetaminophen (Tylenol), ibuprofen (Advil), naproxen sodium (Aleve), and aspirin, can help to reduce the pain you feel. However, tell your doctor what you are using as some of these should not be taken if your doctor has prescribed a nonsteroid anti-inflammatory drug (NSAIDs).

Physical Therapy

Physical therapy programs designed by physiatrists and physical therapists are often useful and may include various specific exercises, galvanic ultrasound, stretch techniques, manual manipulation, myofascial release techniques, traction modalities (e.g., Pronex device), and sustained natural apophyseal glide (SNAG) mobilization techniques.

Natural Cures

Hydrotherapy.   When you first notice neck or back pain, it's important to treat the pain immediately with compresses of either ice or heat on the injured site—whichever brings you the most relief. I recommend that patients use ice compresses for at least ten minutes each waking hour for the first seventy-eight hours after injury for optimal relief.

Many women also find excellent neck or back pain relief with applications of moist heat on the painful area. You may use a moist heating pad; a warm, damp towel; or a hydrocollator pack. Or try standing or sitting on a stool in the shower and letting warm water hit the injured area on the neck or back. A sitz bath—a warm water bath that covers the lower abdomen, hips, and buttocks—or a Jacuzzi bath are other enjoyable ways to find pain relief.

If you wish to try moist heat, do so twice a day or more, for at least twenty minutes each time. You may want to alternate the ice compresses with the moist heat for optimal benefit. You may use the moist heat for a few minutes just before and after back exercises, to make them less painful and more effective.

Dietary Supplements.   Ultimately, we'd all like to find relief with natural cures—those therapies that can be administered without a doctor's visit. Some of the most popular include healing herbs such as feverfew, white willow, and devil's claw, which help to reduce inflammation and pain. If nervous tension or disrupted sleep increases the pain, valerian root or natural hormone melatonin may help to calm you down and increase sound sleep. Many women also find excellent relief with natural supplements such as SAM-e, fish oil capsules, and glucosamine and chondroitin sulfate, if osteoarthritis is the cause of neck or back pain. If you are seeing a doctor, make sure he or she knows about natural remedies you may have chose to try.

Exercise

While mobilization is important with neck or back pain, many women say they'd rather rest in bed until the pain ends! Still, regular exercise, which maintains overall conditioning and flexibility, is important for resolving pain. Over a period of time, exercise will also help you to lose weight or maintain a normal weight, which will ease back pain.

If your pain stems from an injury and you are confined to bed rest for two or three days, you should begin to exercise while lying down on the bed, then advance to a standing position. You can try some of the safe stretching exercises described in Step 4, and then walk around your house for periods of five to ten minutes until you have good pain relief. Increase exercise as your pain diminishes.

When you are pain-free, try a yoga posture called the cobra, described on page 194. This posture helps to alleviate the pressure on the lower back.

Healing Nutrients

Antioxidants and Phytochemicals.   Foods high in antioxidants and phytochemicals boost the healing power of your immune system, which is vital to help you stay well. Vitamin C, a key antioxidant, is a major player in protecting the body from the formation of free radicals. Free radicals cause cell damage and impair the immune system. When you add vitamin C supplementation or boost your food intake of vitamin C (and other antioxidants), you can increase the free radical scavenging process. In addition, a diet high in calcium and vitamin D can help keep your bones strong and keep osteo-porosis—and the painful fractures—at bay. Eating foods that decrease inflammation, such as pineapple or papaya, may help to ease nagging back or neck pain. Taking essential fatty acids (fish oil, flaxseed oil, evening primrose oil, or borage) and vitamin E can give a boost to tissue healing. Be sure to use top-quality vitamin E, either the d-alpha or mixed tocopheral types.

Eat Fish.   Researchers believe that eating high-fat fish such as tuna, mackerel, cod, or salmon—all rich in omega-3 fatty acids—enables the body to make more products that tend to decrease inflammation. Besides omega-3s, salmon is rich in calcium, magnesium, some carotenoids, complete proteins, and B vitamins. Vitamin B6 supports immune function, as discussed in Step 5.

Lose Weight.   Staying at a normal weight is very important in alleviating back pain. To understand how increased weight affects your back, imagine wearing a coat that weighs twenty, thirty, or fifty pounds. This additional weight affects the way you walk, sit, and move during daily activities. If you are overweight, your back pain may improve from weight loss even without medications or other more invasive therapies.

A study published in the December 2001 issue of the journal *Spine* reiterated that people with large abdomens need to get in shape to help alleviate back pain. Abdominal muscles are crucial for stabilizing your posture, and having a protruding tummy is like holding a large box in front of you. To compensate for the extra girth, you have to use more back muscles. This can throw your body out of alignment, causing back strain and injury.

Ask your doctor or a nutritionist for more information on eating healthily to lose weight. I've outlined a recommended weight loss and nutrition program for women with chronic pain in Step 5. Also focus on exercises in Step 4 to tighten up flabby abdominal muscles.

Mind/Body Exercise

Avoid stressful situations, as stress may lower your immune defenses. Learn how to work periods of time-out or relaxation into your daily routine to ease tension and give your body time to recover. You will notice a dramatic difference in the pain you feel.

Distraction is also an excellent tool for easing chronic neck or back pain, and mind/body exercises can help you achieve that. Some of the most popular ones include biofeedback, relaxation response, deep abdominal breathing, visualization or guided imagery, music therapy, and prayer or meditation—all discussed in Step 6. Cognitive behavioral techniques employed by behavioral medicine specialists may also be useful.

Bodywork and Massage

There are many touch therapies that help boost endorphins, brain chemicals that have an opioid effect in the body, as well as speed healing by increasing blood flow. Hands-on therapies are known to improve functioning, as well as lessen pain. In fact, massage therapy may give the most relief for back pain, according to a study published in *The Archives of Internal Medicine*. In this study, back pain patients given massage therapy reported less disability and fewer symptoms after ten weeks than patients who were given traditional Chinese acupuncture or a book and videotapes on managing back pain. The massage group also used the least medication and had the lowest costs of subsequent care.

Still, acupuncture has been found to give excellent relief for both neck and back pain. In fact, a large study from Germany found that more than 50 percent of patients surveyed received relief from pain in less than two weeks of treatment. Researchers believe that acupuncture may alter brain chemistry by changing the release of neurotransmitters and brain hormones in a good way. (However, results from acupuncture may be operator-dependent, as discussed in Step 7.)

Other types of hands-on therapies for back pain include acupressure, shiatsu, Swedish massage, deep muscle massage, and chiropractic.

High-Tech Solutions

Other noninvasive pain therapies include injections, nerve blocks, spinal drug delivery system using a pump to deliver pain relief medications, spinal cord stimulation, the use of a Pronex device (a lightweight pneumatic device that can be used at home for cervical traction effects), transcutaneous electrical nerve stimulation (TENS), and ultrasound, all explained in Step 8. Work with your doctor to find which treatment works best for your type of back or neck pain; in many cases, a combination of therapies will help resolve pain and give you back quality of life.

For some women with chronic or long-lasting, progressive back pain or neurologic deficits such as foot drop, surgery may be the appropriate treatment option as it allows you to become active again. However, I usually only recommend surgery as a last resort when patients cannot manage their symptoms using more conservative nonsurgical treatment.

If disc problems are the source of your back pain, there are newer, more interventional (aggressive) procedures discussed in Step 8 that might help. Although these procedures are not considered "full-blown" surgery, they are relatively new and do not have large multi-center outcome studies demonstrating significant efficacy. However, they may work for some people. Talk to your doctor about your pain problem to see if these interventional procedures may help.

When to Call the Doctor

When your neck or back pain occurs for the first time, consult your doctor for a diagnosis of the problem; if the pain lasts for more than a few days, it is even more important to seek help, as the pain can interfere with your work, activities, relationships, and sleep. Pain that is severe and unending should alert you to seek immediate medical evaluation. Call your doctor if you experience any of the following symptoms:

- Pain that is worse when you cough or sneeze
- Pain or numbness that travels down one or both legs or arms
- Pain that awakens you from sleep
- Difficulty passing urine or having a bowel movement
- Partial or total loss of bladder or bowel control
- Weight loss
- Fever
- Pain in a bone or in the abdomen

These symptoms may be early indicators of serious nerve damage or other serious medical problems, such as arthritis, osteoporosis, cancer, or diseases of internal organs. Sometimes neck or jaw pain can be the first sign of a heart attack; don't take this lightly when you first experience pain. Early diagnosis and treatment will help you get the best results.

CHAPTER FOUR

Gynecologic Pain

Bearing pain has often seemed the duty of women throughout the history of humankind. Consider our grandmothers and the millions of other women who suffered with the pain of childbirth, most without pain-relieving medications or alternative therapies. Or think about the more than 40 percent of all American women today who suffer monthly with debilitating menstrual cramps. More than 10 percent of these women are incapacitated for one to three days each month because of excruciating pain. And what about the chronic back and abdominal pain during the premenstrual period—that time of the month when hormones wreak havoc with the female body? There is no doubt that gynecologic pain has touched the lives of almost all women at some time.

Still, I find it difficult to believe that while almost all women have experienced pain with their menstrual cycle, only half have ever discussed it with their doctors. A recent national online survey conducted by the National Women's Health Resource Center (NWHRC) found that many women don't talk to their doctors because most of them don't believe that doctors can actually do something about the pain.

If your doctor ignores your pain, then find a health care professional who will listen and act aggressively. There are plenty of available options—medical and complementary—to help you resolve pain. Let's evaluate some of the most common causes of gynecologic pain, along with specific recommendations to put a halt to the pain.

Menstrual Cramps

Janie said she spent "half her life" lying on the couch with a heating pad and the other half anticipating the bloating and cramping from her menstrual period. This twenty-nine-year-old flight attendant felt like nothing she tried seemed to help. Her menstrual pain almost cost her an excellent career, as she would miss days at a time from work—until she started taking Vioxx, a Cox-2 inhibitor (Super Aspirin), along with a long-acting progestin called medroxyprogesterone acetate. The Super Aspirin reduced the production of prostaglandins, resulting in less pain, while the progestin prevented ovulation (the monthly release of an egg), giving Janie lighter, more regular menstrual periods and reduced cramping.

What You Might Feel: Signs and Symptoms

Almost every woman has experienced the debilitating pain of menstrual cramps (dysmenorrhea). Mild to intense abdominal cramping typically begins within twenty-four hours of the start of your period and continues for several days. Most women who suffer with cramps also experience aching in the upper thighs, along with lower back pain, bloating and abdominal distension, nausea, diarrhea, and fatigue, among other symptoms. Some women even experience *mittelschmerz*, mid-cycle abdominal pain felt at the time of ovulation.

What Causes Menstrual Cramps?

Menstrual cramps are generally categorized as "primary dysmenorrhea," which is caused by the elevated production of prostaglandins, hormones produced by the uterus that cause it to contract. When you have strong uterine contractions, the blood supply to the uterus is momentarily shut down, depriving the uterine muscle of oxygen and setting up the cycle of menstrual contractions and pain. Some studies show that women with severe menstrual cramps have stronger uterine contractions than other women do when giving birth.

If you suffer with more severe menstrual cramping called "secondary dysmenorrhea," it may be the result of a more serious gynecological problem, such as a uterine fibroid tumor, endometriosis or pelvic infection.

ARE YOU AT RISK?

Risk Factors for Primary Dysmenorrhea
- Never having been pregnant
- Menstrual periods longer than five days
- Obesity
- Cigarette smoking
- Alcohol use
- Family history

Risk Factors for Secondary Dysmenorrhea
- Endometriosis
- Pelvic infection
- Intrauterine device
- Uterine fibroid tumor
- Sexually transmitted diseases

How Menstrual Pain Is Diagnosed

To diagnose the cause of your cramps, your doctor will first perform a pelvic examination with a Pap smear, a test for distinguishing normal from abnormal cells of the cervix. If cervical abnormalities or cancer is detected early, it is usually treatable. Your doctor will determine uterine size and mobility, and look for any unusual redness, tenderness, inflammation, or enlargement. Your doctor may find specific medical problems such as uterine malformations or genital infections and be able treat these early on. Blood tests will be done to see if you are anemic or have an infection or other signs of illness.

CHRONIC PELVIC PAIN

Chronic pelvic pain is another common complaint, particularly from women of childbearing age. This pain could be gynecological in nature, or it may stem from irritable bowel syndrome (IBS), interstitial cystitis (IC), or pelvic floor myofascial syndrome. This continuous or intermittent pelvic pain may last for months with no known cause or cure.

Treating Menstrual Cramps

Medication

Nonsteroid Anti-inflammatory Drugs.   Over-the-counter nonsteroid anti-inflammatory drugs (NSAIDs), such as ibuprofen (Advil), are the gold standard in relieving most cases of menstrual cramps. NSAIDs work by blocking the effects of prostaglandins, the chemicals that cause inflammation, pain, and swelling. These medications should be taken with food about two or three days before the start of your period to get the most benefit, and should be taken around the clock, as directed on the label.

NSAIDs work best when preventing pain, and that's why treating pain before it starts will help keep your cramps minimal. (Most of the prostaglandins are released during the first forty-eight hours of your menstrual period.) However, use caution with NSAIDs, as they can cause stomach upset or even ulcers.

Cox-2 Inhibitors.   The new Super Aspirins, Cox-2 inhibitors such as valdecoxib (Bextra), rofecoxib (Vioxx), and celecoxib (Celebrex), are now approved for treating menstrual pain. These prescription medications work in the same way as NSAIDs to block prostaglandin production and reduce inflammation and pain, yet they are easily tolerated by the gastrointestinal system.

Oral Contraceptives.   If NSAIDs or Super Aspirins fail to stop your menstrual cramping, ask your doctor about oral contraceptives. Most women with mild to moderate cramping (primary dysmenorrhea) who take birth control pills have less pain, lighter periods, and regular menstrual cycles. Also consider taking a nonsteroid anti-inflammatory drug (NSAIDs) along with the oral contraceptive to get the most benefit in decreasing inflammation and pain.

Progestasert IUD.   In most cases, intrauterine devices (IUDs) can actually cause more pain and a heavier menstrual flow. But some women have found success with the Progestasert IUD, which releases a tiny amount of progesterone into the uterus and may help to stop cramping. Ask your doctor if this may alter your menstrual pain.

Natural Cures

Plant Medicines.   There are plenty of botanical (plant) medicines, such as yarrow used in hot tea, that have been used throughout history to treat painful menstrual cramps. Ginger has antispasmodic properties and can quell nausea and gastrointestinal upset associated with the menstrual period. While not substantiated by science, some of these herbal therapies, including the following (discussed in Step 3), appear to have some therapeutic influence in easing menstrual cramps: fennel, sage, Dong Quai, red clover, chamomile, raspberry leaf, boswellia, vitex chaste tree, gingko biloba.

Moist Heat Reduces Inflammation.   Most of my patients find excellent relief from menstrual cramps with a moist heating pad, a combination of hydrotherapy and heat. In a study published in March 2001 in the *Journal of Obstetrics and Gynecology*, pain researchers found that heat may help ease menstrual cramps as much as ibuprofen. While doctors are not sure as to the pain-reducing mechanism of heat, we do know that heat is a vasodilator that increases blood flow, and it counteracts the activity of hormones that cause the uterus to relax.

Exercise

Just when I told you to get relief by lying on your couch, clutching a heating pad, I'm now going to give you a bit of different advice: to end menstrual cramps, get up and stretch. Move around more. Yes, exercise! Exercise is proven to improve blood flow throughout the abdomen and to increase endorphins, pain-relieving substances naturally produced by your body. Some women find that sexual activity—a type of exercise—relieves menstrual cramping and nagging backaches. Having an orgasm helps by dispersing the blood that is congested in the pelvic area. (Note: If you have endometriosis, this may worsen your menstrual pain.)

Healing Nutrients

Low-Fat, High-Fiber.   Eating to decrease pain can be quite pleasurable, especially if you prefer low-fat, high-fiber vegetarian cuisine. A recent study published in the journal *Obstetrics and Gynecology* concluded that women who ate such a diet had significant reduction in the duration and intensity of menstrual pain. They were also more likely to lose weight and lower their Body Mass Index (explained on page 202), while on the low-fat, high-fiber diet than during the placebo phase of the study.

The study diet was associated with significantly higher serum levels of sex-hormone-binding globulin and lower serum estrogen levels. Bile contains estrogen conjugates and a diet high in plant fiber increases the amount of estrogen excreted in feces. The ensuing decline in estrogen, together with increased sex-hormone-binding globulin, may reduce the endometrial production of prostaglandin-producing tissues and help to alleviate painful menstrual cramps.

Substitute Beans and Legumes for Protein.   Beans, such as soy, adzuki, kidney, and pinto, and legumes like red lentils and yellow split peas, are also effective in balancing estrogen. Besides being excellent sources of protein, they contain plant compounds called isoflavones (specifically genistein and daidzein), which are known to be estrogen-mimics.

Focus on Specific Nutrients.   Be sure to include specific pain-defying nutrients in your daily diet. These vitamins and minerals have been shown to possibly decrease inflammation and pain: omega-3 fatty acids, calcium, magnesium, vitamin E, vitamin B6.

Fatty Acids May Give Relief.   Flaxseed is another food that may help ease menstrual cramps if taken over a period of several months. Flaxseed is a megasource for alpha-linolenic acid, the plant version of omega-3 fatty acids. These tiny black seeds are also high in lignans, a type of fiber found to help estrogen-related conditions. You can sprinkle flaxseed on yogurt or cereal, or use it in smoothies. Flaxseed oil is available at most health food stores in liquid or capsule form.

Evening primrose oil is a supplement some women find helpful in easing cramps. It contains gamma-linolenic acid (GLA), an essential fatty acid that the body converts to a substance called prostaglandin E1, which may possess anti-inflammatory properties.

Mind/Body Exercises

When patients tell me that menstrual pain is much worse on days when they are totally stressed out, I explain how relaxation is a vital part of relieving pain. In fact, I've seen many women who were able to function quite normally even with menstrual cramps once they learned how to totally relax their bodies and minds. While most studies are not conclusive on the benefits of mind/body therapy to the gynecological system, we do know that an excess of the stress hormone cortisol throws your other hormones into chaos, resulting in disrupted menstrual cycles in many women. Also, depression interferes with all sorts of hormones that may adversely affect ovulation. It makes good sense that learning to relax your body before you encounter a crisis or stressor is the best way to protect yourself from future hormone havoc, including the resulting cramps.

Some of the best relaxation tools to ease cramping include deep abdominal breathing, visualization, deep muscle relaxation, and meditation.

Bodywork and Massage

A deep muscle massage can help to relax your back and abdomen during a painful menstrual period. Acupuncture is also a useful, non-pharmacological method for treating cramps, as it helps to block pain impulses. Acupressure, as discussed on page 239–240, and self-massage are helpful in relaxing painful muscles and can be done in the privacy of your own home. Use a soothing aromatherapy oil to get even more sensory benefits.

High-Tech Solutions

For women who have menstrual pain so severe it keeps them from being active and doing their daily activities, I've found that wearing a TENS unit (a small electrical device that interferes with pain signals as they travel to the brain) can often help lessen the cramps. The TENS unit alters the body's ability to receive or perceive pain signals and allows you to move about your day without having to sit with a heating pad to get relief. Caution: Make certain you are not pregnant before using this.

When to Call the Doctor

If your cramps suddenly worsen and are painful for longer than normal, or if you have sudden, severe pain, heavy bleeding, or a fever of more than 100 degrees F., call your doctor. These may be signs of a more serious problem that needs to be evaluated and treated.

SOOTHING SMOOTHIE

This soothing smoothie is high in protein as well as essential pain-reducing nutrients, making it a healthy way to start your active day.

Ingredients

½ cup soymilk
½ cup nonfat yogurt
½ cup calcium enriched skim milk
1 cup fresh fruit (pineapple, strawberries, blueberries)
½ banana
1 tablespoon flaxseed oil (or freshly ground flaxseed)
1 teaspoon flavored extract
honey or sugar to taste
2 ice cubes

Put all ingredients in a blender and process until smooth. Makes 1 serving.

Note: If you cannot tolerate soy, use 1/2 cup calcium-fortified orange juice instead of soymilk.

Minimize PMS with Natural Therapies

Millions of women suffer from premenstrual syndrome which includes breast tenderness, cramping, and backache. While there is no known cause or cure for PMS, researchers believe that normal cyclical changes in a woman's hormones may interact with neurotransmitters, including serotonin. This may result in the mood swings, pain, and other physical symptoms of PMS. Consider the following natural therapies, discussed fully in my 8-step program, to minimize pain and other PMS symptoms:

- Try St. John's wort to ease anxiety, but check with your doctor if you are taking any other medications to avoid herb-drug interactions.
- Take evening primrose oil to decrease inflammation.
- Apply moist heat to the painful areas.
- Exercise regularly to decrease fluid retention and increase sense of well-being.
- Avoid alcohol, as it may compound feelings of depression before your period.
- Avoid caffeine before and during your period.
- Reduce salt in your diet to reduce bloating, edema, and fluid weight gain.
- Increase intake of fresh fruits, vegetables, cereals, and grains.
- Drink plenty of liquids.

Endometriosis

Sometimes tagged as "the most underdiagnosed disease of women," endometriosis is often the source of more serious menstrual cramping. Not only can this disease prevent conception, it is frequently the cause of miscarriage or early pregnancy loss.

What You Might Feel: Signs and Symptoms

Because hormones control endometriosis, you may have pelvic pain during certain times of the month such as ovulation and menstruation. Additional symptoms include painful intercourse, painful bowel movements, painful urination, and heavy periods and bleeding between periods.

What Causes Endometriosis?

Endometriosis is thought to be associated with the backflow of menstrual fluid and tissue through the tubes and out into the pelvic cavity (retrograde menstruation). These implantation locations are mostly in the pelvis, but in some cases endometriosis can be found outside the pelvis. The effect on infertility depends upon both how much of the tissue is present, and the location of the tissue. Both factors then influence how much damage is done to the pelvis.

With endometriosis your body produces more prostaglandins, chemicals in the body that cause inflammation and pain. But endometriosis is a progressive disease, only slowing down at pregnancy or menopause.

ARE YOU AT RISK?

Risk Factors for Endometriosis

- Menstrual cycle less than twenty-eight days
- Bleeding more than five days
- Painful periods
- Infertility
- Congenital abnormality of the uterus
- Abnormally tight cervical opening
- Family history

How Endometriosis Is Diagnosed

If you have symptoms of spastic colon (irritable bowel syndrome), painful periods, chronic urinary bladder pain, painful intercourse, or an abnormal bleeding pattern, your doctor may suspect endometriosis and start with a complete physical examination, including a pelvic exam and PAP smear, to make the diagnosis. During an exam, your doctor may feel nodules (which are the endometriosis cysts aka endometriomas) along the uterosacral ligaments that attach your cervix to the backbone. Sometimes clinicians can see a cyst which has a "ground glass" appearance of an endometrioma on imaging studies which may increase suspicion of endometriosis.

Endometriosis may occur anywhere in the body and is usually "picked up" by an ultrasound scan. However, magnetic resonance imaging (MRI) may have advantages, detecting small cysts in the abdominal wall, ovaries, subperitoneum, bladder, and rectum. Endoscopic ultrasound and CT (virtual) colonoscopy may be helpful for detection of sigmoid endometriosis.

While your doctor may determine that you have endometriosis from evaluating your medical history, the only sure way to diagnose this condition is by surgery, specifically laparoscopy, which your doctor can explain. Ultrasound and laparoscopy are also important in ruling out any malignancies, such as ovarian cancer, that may mimic endometriosis. Once the implants and scar tissue (adhesions) are found in moderate or severe endometriosis, the surgeon will proceed to treat this. However, if your condition is mild, it may just require a very careful inspection of the pelvis by an experienced laparoscopic surgeon. Keep in mind that just because it is mild does not mean that endometriosis is not a cause for your menstrual pain.

Treating Endometriosis Pain

Medication

Nonsteroid Anti-inflammatory Drugs.   Right now, the treatment of endometriosis is controversial, with the choices of medical therapy, surgery, or a combination of the two. First, as with menstrual cramps, nonsteroid anti-inflammatory drugs (NSAIDs) block prostaglandins, and are effective in relieving pain in some women. The new Cox-2 inhibitors (Celebrex, Bextra, Vioxx) also block prostaglandin production and may help end pain without stomach upset. If these drugs fail to relieve the pain, your doctor may give you narcotic medications.

GnRH Analogs.   Other medications effective in relieving pain include GnRH analogs or GnRH-A (Lupron, Synarel, and Zoladex) and Danazol. GnRH-A works by turning off the ovaries, which generate most of the hormone estrogen. Estrogen acts as a "fertilizer" for endometriosis, so reducing its production reduces the stimulation for endometriosis to grow.

While the GnRH analogs treat endometriosis, the side effects are similar to menopause, with hot flashes, vaginal dryness, insomnia, and bone loss. A newer long-term treatment program involves adding back small amounts of estrogen and progestins to reduce these symptoms and at the same time to keep the endometriosis in check. Danazol has been shown to have a lethal effect on endometriosis cells. But the side effects are not pleasant, including weight gain, acne, abnormal hair growth, and occasionally mood changes. Experimental hormonal therapies called aromatase inhibitors act similarly to Danazol and are now being studied for treating endometriosis.

Oral Contraceptives.   Other medical therapies, including continuous oral contraceptives, may retard the development of endometriosis, but they are usually not enough to treat the disease.

Natural Cures

Moist Heat.   As with menstrual cramps, moist heat applied to the abdomen and back can help to reduce inflammation and congestion. You may use a moist heating pad, warm sitz bath, or sit in a heated 104-degree Jacuzzi for a limited time to relax your entire body. (If you are pregnant, do not sit in hot baths or Jacuzzis.)

Herbal Relief.   Some patients find relief with soothing herbal teas, including chamomile, valerian, and raspberry leaf. Others find that ginseng helps to balance hormones, resulting in less pain during the menstrual cycle.

Exercise

Choose Low-Intensity Activities.   Low-intensity exercise, such as walking or stretching, may help to boost blood flow and reduce the cramping you feel. Avoid high-intensity exercise as it may increase pain.

Yoga.   Many women with endometriosis find that yoga (see chapter 12) helps ease the intense pain and enables them to focus on thoughts that are more positive as well.

Healing Nutrients

Follow the same low-fat, high-fiber diet recommended for regular menstrual cramps (see page 48). Add fish high in omega-3 fatty acids to your diet, including mackerel, salmon, herring, sardines, sable fish (black cod), anchovies, and tuna.

Preliminary studies show that soybean and avocado oil may be helpful in reducing inflammation. You may want to incorporate these foods in your daily diet to see if they help you feel less pain.

Mind/Body Exercises

Having any chronic health problem can leave you feeling angry and depressed. But with endometriosis, the consequences, such as infertility or miscarriage, can also be devastating. That's why understanding your emotions and channeling these in a positive way may help you to feel more upbeat as your doctor works with you on treatment. Any of the mind/body exercises discussed in Step 6 can be helpful for de-stressing and relaxation.

Bodywork and Massage

With a chronic problem like endometriosis, you may try regular weekly massages to relieve tension and stimulate the release of the body's natural opioidlike endorphins. Some women find acupuncture treatments very helpful in easing the ongoing pain and discomfort. I'd recommend a minimum of six to eight treatments with a licensed acupuncture professional to see if this works for you.

High-Tech Solutions

As with easing other menstrual cramps, a TENS machine, a small hand-held machine described in Step 8, stimulates acupuncture points electrically and has been a useful adjunct for the treatment of the pain for some women. Still, in severe cases, surgery is the only way to end the pain of endometriosis, however, this is usually able to be accomplished using laparosopic techniques. This invasive procedure can be done by laser (evaporation), harmonic scalpel (cutting), or electrocautery (burning). The important goal is to eliminate as much of the "problem" tissue as possible without causing harm to pelvic organs, which is best done by a surgeon experienced in endometrial surgery. (Experience combined with appropriate extensive laparoscopic techniques are key.)

When to Call the Doctor

If your pain or bleeding worsens, see your doctor for an immediate evaluation.

Pelvic Inflammatory Disease

Sometimes endometriosis is mistaken for pelvic inflammatory disease (PID), infections or inflammations that have the potential for permanently scarring the reproductive tract—the uterus, ovaries, or fallopian tubes—leading to infertility.

Symptoms of PID may be mild and easily dismissed as an intestinal bug. Or, the symptoms may be severe enough to require hospitalization. The most common signs and symptoms include:

- Abdominal/pelvic discomfort
- Painful urination
- Pain during intercourse
- Abnormal bleeding
- Vaginal discharge with an unpleasant odor
- Fever and chills

The vast majority of PID stems from sexually transmitted diseases (STDs). The only method of transmission of gonorrhea or chlamydia is by recent sexual contact with an infected person, as the organisms do not live outside the body. Another common cause of PID is a "mixed infection" usually arising from contamination by microorganisms from the intestine or vagina. This form of PID may have no relation to multiple partners.

Less common causes of PID include a ruptured cyst or appendix, pelvic surgery, or a bowel injury. Risk factors include the following:

- Female under age twenty-five
- More than one sex partner
- Have had STDs or a prior case of PID
- Your partner has had more than one sexual partner

If you have symptoms of PID, see your doctor. The organisms that cause chlamydia and gonorrhea infection are easily identified on tests of cervical cells, and other blood tests are done to check the severity of infection.

Treatment for PID is antibiotics (often more than one kind over a period of three to four weeks) and bed rest. If the infection is severe, intravenous antibiotics may need to be given in a hospital. If left untreated, pelvic infections may leave residual scarring that will hamper fertility. The good news is that pelvic infection and its scarring can be prevented by aggressive antibiotic therapy.

VULVAR PAIN

Vulvovaginitis may be due to allergic reaction (contact vaginitis), infection (bacterial, parasitic, fungal), or hypoestrogenism (atrophic). Symptoms include burning, discomfort, painful intercourse, and vaginal discharge. It is important to localize the pain in order to arrive at a diagnosis and proper treatment.

Uterine Fibroids

Uterine fibroids (*myomasor leiomyomas*) are the most common tumors in the female reproductive system. It is estimated that four out of five women over the age of thirty-five have uterine fibroids.

What You Might Feel: Signs and Symptoms

Many fibroids cause nothing more than mild pelvic pressure. However other common symptoms include:

- Pelvic pain
- Painful periods
- Pelvic pressure or fullness
- Heavy periods
- Frequent or difficult urination
- Chronic back pain

What Causes Uterine Fibroids?

Each fibroid begins its development as a single muscle cell; for unknown reasons, it begins to duplicate. While it is not known what causes fibroids to grow, these tumors are under the control of estrogen and progesterone, the principal ovarian hormones. After menopause, when the estrogen levels fall, fibroids decrease in size.

ARE YOU AT RISK?

Age (by age 35, 4 out of 5 women have fibroid tumors)
Oral contraceptive use
Race (African Americans have increased risk)

How Are Uterine Fibroids Diagnosed?

Your doctor may suspect a fibroid tumor during a pelvic examination. Ultrasound scan is an excellent diagnostic tool for fibroids. In select cases, more extensive imaging with MRI may be necessary.

Treating Fibroid Tumor Pain

Medication

Treatment may vary from medication to surgery to simply observing the tumor. Nonsteroidal anti-inflammatory drugs (NSAIDs), such as ibuprofen, can help to stop pain and cramping and may decrease blood loss. The hormonal treatment Danazol may help to control heavy menstrual flow. Since fibroids are controlled by ovarian hormones, other drugs, known as gonadotropin-releasing hormone (GnRH) agonists may be used to shrink fibroids by reducing the amount of estrogen in your body. The reduction in hormonal stimulation may stop fibroid growth and often results in their shrinkage. Unfortunately, although the chemicals may reduce the fibroid size by 50 percent, it will quickly return when the suppressive therapy is stopped.

Natural Cures

There are no known natural cures for fibroid tumors, although the exercise, diet, mind/body exercises, and bodyworks given for menstrual cramps will enable you to decrease the pain and inflammation you normally feel during your period (see pages 47–51).

High-Tech Solutions

Submucosal fibroids, those adjacent to the endometrium, may be surgically removed by hysteroscopy. Sometimes a procedure called a myomectomy may be used, which helps preserve fertility. This procedure is performed through an abdomen incision, a laparotomy, or laparoscopy. Once the fibroid is removed, the surrounding muscle is usually closed with sutures, and the area forms a scar. This scar may not expand as well as the muscle during pregnancy and could result in a uterine rupture. If you've had a fibroid removed and plan on getting pregnant, ask your doctor about the possibilities of a cesarean section.

UTERINE FIBROID EMBOLIZATION (UFE)

While in many parts of the United States hysterectomy or myomectomy is still the only treatment option for uterine fibroids, a relatively new treatment called uterine fibroid embolization (UFE) is proving to be a quick and safe option for women with symptomatic fibroids who do not want to undergo surgery. This outpatient procedure is particularly effective in relieving excessive menstrual bleeding caused by the condition.

In UFE, doctors make a small incision in the leg. Using X ray guidance, a catheter is manipulated through blood vessels until the uterine artery is reached. Then doctors inject small particles, the size of grains of sand, into the uterine arteries. The blood supply that feeds uterine fibroids is blocked (embolized), the fibroids shrink, and symptoms improve or disappear. UFE is an extremely safe and minimally invasive procedure that is performed by vascular interventional radiologists under local anesthesia.

Fibrocystic Breast Changes (FBC)

Almost all women have experienced breast pain and immediately feared the worst—cancer. Yet in most cases, the cause of breast pain is hormonal, as about 60 percent of women ages thirty to fifty-five have experienced this sensitivity or tenderness during the second half of their menstrual cycle. During this time progesterone is dominant; the lobules at the ends of the mammary glands start to multiply and surrounding breast tissues swell.

While not really a "disease," fibrocystic breast change (cystic mastitis) forms noncancerous cysts that are usually harmless. Yet in some cases they may be cancerous, which means that early detection and diagnosis of this condition is important.

What You Might Feel: Signs and Symptoms

With fibrocystic breast changes, you will feel swelling, pain, and lumpiness in both breasts, usually around the time of your menstrual period because of fluid retention. Sometimes you may feel a sharp pain or burning sensation in the breasts. Most of the symptoms resolve after menopause with the decline in estrogen, unless you are taking hormone replacement therapy.

What Causes Fibrocystic Breast Changes?

The primary contributing factor to fibrocystic breast changes is the normal hormonal variation during your menstrual cycle. As the body prepares to menstruate, hormones stimulate fluids to build up and form cysts, fluid-filled sacs in the breast that fell like small knots. These cysts then irritate the fibrous breast tissue, resulting in tender or painful and easily felt lumps. After menstruation, irritation diminishes but fibroidal cysts don't disappear.

ARE YOU AT RISK?

Childbearing years
Irregular menstrual cycle
Hormonal abnormalities (diabetes, thyroid disease)

How Are Fibrocystic Breast Changes Diagnosed?

Monthly self-examination of your breasts will help you know how your breasts normally look and feel and allow you to detect changes. Fibrocystic breasts changes can feel lumpy, irregular, or like tiny beads, usually in the upper quadrant of the breast (near your armpit). Regular breast examinations by a doctor also are recommended as fibrocystic lumps can make breast cancer difficult to detect. Depending on the features of the lump, your doctor may order other diagnostic tests, such as an ultrasound of the breasts, a mammogram, or even a tissue biopsy to help determine the cause.

Treating Fibrocystic Breast Pain

Medication

Nonsteroid anti-inflammatory drugs (NSAIDs) are useful in alleviating the nagging pain of fibrocystic breast changes. Some women
who have irregular menstrual cycles, one of the risk factors for this
condition, find relief with low-dose birth control pills. Diuretics are
also used with success, as they eliminate excess fluid. In severe cases,
Tamoxifen (a selective estrogen receptor modulator, or SERM) is
used to block the action of estrogen, resulting in fewer breast lumps.
Ask your doctor about this medication.

Natural Cures

Support Your Breasts.   Wear a good-fitting bra to support your
breasts. Some women find excellent relief with regular applications
of heat compresses on the breast to relieve swelling.

Cut Out Caffeine.   According to a study published in the October
2001 issue of *Fertility and Sterility*, researchers concluded that women
who drink the most coffee have higher levels of estradiol, a naturally
occurring form of estrogen, during the early follicular phase, or days
one to five of the menstrual cycle. In the study, done at Brigham and
Women's Hospital in Boston, researchers noted that women who consumed at least 500 milligrams of caffeine daily, the equivalent of four
or five cups of coffee, had nearly 70 percent more estrogen during the
early follicular phase than women consuming no more than 100 milligrams of caffeine daily, or less than one cup of coffee. Because estrogen fuels fibrocystic breast conditions, substitute any caffeine with
another drink to see if this may help you lessen pain. For the same reason, avoid chocolate or any medication that contains caffeine.

Exercise

Exercise can help keep your hormones balanced and your body
working at peak performance level. Be sure to wear a good support
bra when you exercise to avoid injury to the breasts.

Healing Nutrients

Try to incorporate some of the following healing substances and
their primary sources:

- Polyphenols, which are found in vegetables, fruits, and green tea
- Isothiocyanates and indoles, two phytochemicals found in broccoli, cauliflower, bok choy, brussels sprouts, mustard greens, radishes, turnips, and other cruciferous vegetables
- Bioflavonoids, which have an antioxidant effect in the body, found in red grapes, bilberries, strawberries, and citrus fruits
- Terpenoids, healing phytochemicals found in citrus fruits
- Isoflavones, plantlike estrogenic compound found in soybeans

Supplement Your Diet.   Vitamin E, a powerful antioxidant important to the body for the maintenance of cell membranes, is thought to help reduce the pain of fibrocystic breast changes. Studies reveal that vitamin E helps stimulate the function of T-cells, which are important fighters of the immune system.

Mind/Body Exercise

As with any chronic problem, staying focused on the moment instead of worrying about the future helps you maintain a sense of balance. Learn the relaxation response (page 227–229) and use this anytime you become overwhelmed from life's stressors.

Bodywork and Massage

Swedish massage can help you relax no matter what crisis you may be experiencing. If fibrocystic breast condition causes you unnecessary symptoms, schedule regular times for massage so you can cope best with the intrusion of chronic pain.

High-Tech Solutions

There is no recommended high-tech solution for fibrocystic breast changes. Treatment is directed as alleviating or reducing symptoms.

When to Call the Doctor

Any time you have an unusual lump or feeling in the breast, call your doctor for an evaluation. Most of the time, it is not serious. Nevertheless, in the case of breast cancer, early detection allows early treatment when it is most successful.

HERPES AND PAIN

Herpes, caused by a virus called *herpes simplex*, is spread by skin-to-skin contact during genital, oral, or anal sex. The symptoms of genital herpes include many painful sores on the genital area, fever, enlarged lymph nodes in the groin area, burning on urination, headache, and flulike symptoms. A first outbreak can last several weeks. Subsequent outbreaks occur as frequently as several times a year. While about 70 percent of the 40 million Americans with genital herpes have no symptoms at all, for those who do suffer an outbreak the pain can be unbearable. An active outbreak during the rupture of membranes or at the time of delivery can be a life-threatening condition for your newborn. It is important that your doctor know of previous herpes infections.

CHAPTER FIVE

Migraine and Headache

There's nothing like a pounding headache to make you seek refuge in a dark, quiet room and hide from the world. If you suffer with chronic headache pain, you have company: More than 45 million Americans have chronic headache pain from migraine, tension, or cluster headaches. Women suffer headaches more frequently than men, perhaps because of variations in the chemical called serotonin, which plays a role in pain and depression. When estrogen levels plummet, levels of serotonin change as well.

Whether you suffer with migraines, tension, or sinus headaches, or headaches from arthritis or jaw pain, all headaches have one central thread that weaves them together: inner and/or outer triggers cause the body to react with pain that is felt in the head. These triggers may stem from foods, tobacco, chemicals, stress, environment, and your hormones, among other things, and the triggers may vary from one woman to the next.

No matter what triggers your headache, it's important to find what works to stop the pain before it overwhelms your life. Let's look at some of the most common headaches women experience and how the 8-step holistic program can help relieve them.

RED FLAG!

If your headache is severe or persistent, you should seek medical advice, as it may be the first sign of a more serious problem. Fortunately, most headaches are not life-threatening, although the pain itself can be very limiting.

Tension Headaches

Janis first started getting tension headaches a few days after her two-year-old daughter, Zoe, had emergency surgery. This twenty-eight-year-old retail buyer was caught off guard when Zoe cut herself with a knife while at her babysitter's home and required outpatient surgery to stop the bleeding in her hand. While the toddler's wound healed beautifully, Janis worried about another accident happening when she left her daughter for the day.

"Since that time, every day around 3:00 P.M. I get this tightness around my forehead that goes to the back of my skull into my neck. It starts very mild and intensifies with each minute—almost feeling like a band that someone continues to tighten until I get home from work, take aspirin, and lie down on my bed for about an hour."

Tension headaches (also called muscle contraction headaches) are the most common types of headaches and happen when the muscles of the neck tighten, causing pain. In Janis's case, the sudden stress of her daughter's injury and surgery, along with fears of it happening again, probably caused her chronic headaches. These episodic tension headaches last from thirty minutes up to seven days or longer, while chronic tension headaches average more than fifteen days each month for more than six months.

What You May Feel: Signs and Symptoms

While both men and women get tension headaches, women are at higher risk. Tension headaches feel like a dull pain in the forehead or back of the head or both, with tightness or pressure in or around the head. The pain may extend over the top of your head to the front near your eyebrows. Some women describe tension headaches as feeling "like you're wearing a hat that's several sizes too small, and it keeps getting smaller, squeezing your head like a vise." You may also have soreness in your shoulders or in the back of your neck. Your neck, jaws, or temporomandibular joint may also hurt if there is tightness of the muscles in these areas.

When this type of headache becomes very frequent or constant, there may also be a great deal of stress present along with depression or other problems. You may have difficulty sleeping at night, eating problems, and fatigue.

What Causes Tension Headache?

As mentioned, tension headaches may be caused by the tightening of the muscles of the neck and head. This is common in times of stress, or when you are tired. Tension headaches may have a genetic link, as it is common for family members to have similar headaches.

ARE YOU AT RISK?

Risk Factors for Tension Headaches

- Stress
- Hunger
- Bad posture
- Sleep deprivation
- Eyestrain
- Age (more common in young adults)

How Are Tension Headaches Diagnosed?

Your doctor will take a complete medical history and do a physical examination. Other causes of headache will be ruled out during this process. In some cases a cranial MRI or cranial CT scan will be used to help make the diagnosis.

WHAT IS THAT PAIN IN YOUR HEAD?

Recurring tension headaches may actually be coming from your cervical spine. In a study published in the June 1997 issue of the *Journal of Manipulative and Physiological Therapy*, researchers concluded that cervicogenic headaches are characterized by pain on one side of the head with associated neck pain on the same side. These headaches may respond to spinal manipulation therapy such as chiropractic.

Vascular or Migraine Headaches

Thirty-six-year old Linda is one of the 28 million Americans who suffer from migraine headaches. As often as four times a week, Linda gets a throbbing feeling in her head, accompanied by overwhelming nausea, vomiting, and sensitivity to light.

When the migraine headache hits, Linda's entire life is put on hold. She calls her sister who lives a few miles away to come get her two preschoolers. Then she pulls down the bedroom shades, and lies in the dark room until the pain and other symptoms subside.

About one in five women suffer from migraine headaches, compared with about one in twenty men. While migraine is the most common type of vascular headache, other types include those caused by high blood pressure (hypertension) and other medical problems. These can include fever, some chemicals, alcohol use, and some foods. Since each of these vascular-type headaches may have treatment available, it is important to first identify the problem. Talk with your physician for advice.

What You May Feel: Signs and Symptoms

Migraine headaches may last from a few hours to days, and can be dull, throbbing, constant, and severe. They may happen only occasionally or may repeat within days. They are most often (but not always) on one side of the head and usually felt in the front or side of the head.

About 20 percent of migraine sufferers have warning signs called "auras," visual sensory disturbances that manifest as flashing lights, stars, distorted shapes, or a "blind" spot and inability to see on one side. The aura is caused by a change in brain activity in the visual cortex section of the brain. Many sufferers get nauseated and vomit with a migraine. Bright light may make the headache much worse. These are all classic warning signs of a migraine and may precede a headache by hours to days.

What Causes Migraines?

While we are not completely sure what causes a migraine headache, it's believed to be the result of a complex cyclic contact between the cranial blood vessels and the trigeminal nerve. A "trigger," such as food, stress, or fatigue, activates neurons that are in charge of releasing a selection of neuropeptides (substance P and neurokinin A). Substance P helps nervous system cells send messages to each other about painful stimuli. It is thought that when substance P levels are elevated in the body, they may produce higher levels of pain. The release of these chemicals causes an increase in blood flow to the brain. The distended blood vessels and the inflammatory response stimulate the trigeminal nerve to send out impulses back to the brain for processing, resulting in a migraine headache.

ARE YOU AT RISK?

Risk Factors for Migraine Headaches

- Genetic predisposition
- Head or neck injury
- Chronic stress
- Trigger foods and beverages
- Skipping meals
- Smoking
- Weather changes
- Bright lights
- Lack of sleep
- Hormone changes (menstruation)

MENSTRUAL MIGRAINE

More than 60 percent of women who suffer with migraine headaches relate them to their menstrual cycle, affirming the link between female hormonal changes and migraine headaches. Interestingly, many women get their first migraine headache at the same time as menarche, and most notice that a migraine attack occurs around their menstrual period. Some migraines occur a few days before, during or immediately after a women's menstrual period, while others occur at mid-cycle during ovulation.

How Are Migraines Diagnosed?

There is no definitive test to distinguish a migraine headache from any other type of head pain, so your doctor will rely on your medical history and physical examination, along with a detailed discussion of symptoms and triggers. Other testing, such as a CT scan, is rarely necessary.

TREATING EYE PAIN

Many headache sufferers, especially those with migraines, also have eye pain. In a study published in the March 2002 issue of *Neurology*, the journal of the American Neurological Association, researchers found that treating inflammation in the eye's trochlea tendon with steroid injections also relieved the headache pain and even prevented a full-blown migraine attack. Talk to your doctor if you have associated eye pain to see if this therapy may be available.

Jaw and Facial Pain

Headaches are common with jaw pain, called temporomandibular joint syndrome (TMJ syndrome). TMJ pain and the TMJ syndrome are common problems that occur usually in younger adults and can mimic a chronic headache.

What You May Feel: Signs and Symptoms

Pain can be felt in the jaw just in front of the ear, or it may be felt over the side of the face and head, and extend to the neck. The pain is often constant and worse with chewing, and there may be a sensation of cracking in the jaw when the mouth is opened. Pain may limit the opening of the jaw, or the jaw may move to one side when it is opened.

What Causes TMJ Pain?

In many cases, dental problems and bite abnormalities can cause TMJ pain. If there is any imbalance in the way your teeth come together, there may be higher pressure in one or both jaws and temporomandibular joints. Or if you are missing teeth on one side, leading to an abnormal chewing motion, it creates higher pressure on the other side of the mouth, leading to TMJ pain.

TMJ pain may be due to arthritis in the temporomandibular joint itself from osteoarthritis or rheumatoid arthritis. If you've had an injury to the jaw, the cartilage of the joint may be damaged, which can result in osteoarthritis of the TMJ.

Ear infections and diseases can also cause TMJ pain, even though the problem is in the ear. In such cases, specific treatment of the ear disease is needed to help the jaw pain.

Stress is a major cause of jaw pain, which can result in even more tension in your face, neck, and jaw. Clenching the teeth during the day or grinding the teeth at night (bruxism) can result from stress and increase the tension on muscles around the jaw. This is a common cause of TMJ pain.

Sometimes TMJ pain is part of a much larger area of pain in the muscles, tendons, and ligaments (soft tissue). With the "soft tissue" pain and fibromyalgia, trigger areas around the jaws, face, and neck may trigger headache pain. In addition, the pain associated with an inadequate blood supply to parts of the heart may occasionally be experienced in the neck and/or jaw.

ARE YOU AT RISK?

Risk Factors for TMJ

- Stress
- Dental problems
- Ear infection
- Arthritis
- Fibromyalgia

Sinus Headache

Headache, particularly pain or pressure around the eyes, across the cheeks and the forehead, is one of the key symptoms of acute or chronic sinusitis. This common headache is associated with a swelling of the membranes that line the sinuses (cavities next to the nasal passages).

What You May Feel: Signs and Symptoms

Sinus pain is often constant, throbbing, and worse when you chew or bend over. Pain can be felt in the jaw just in front of the ear, or it may be felt over the side of the face and head, then extend to the back of the neck, next to the hairline. Other symptoms include:

- Unending or constant pain over cheek or forehead
- Tenderness over the affected sinus and behind the eyes
- A deep dull ache
- Pain that worsens with movements of your head
- Nasal blockage and congestion
- Nasal discharge
- Ear sensations or fullness
- Facial swelling
- Fever (sometimes)

What Causes Sinus Headache?

Any allergic reaction or even a tumor in the sinuses can produce swelling and blockage of the sinuses, causing the headache pain you feel. Although not all pain in the sinus area is directly related to sinus disease, some of the most common causes of pain include:

- *Obstruction.* When the cilia in the nasal passages become damaged or do not work effectively, mucus builds up, causing an obstruction. This obstruction of the sinuses and impacted mucus results in decreased oxygen in your sinus cavities. When the ostia (small opening) in the sinus is blocked, the pressure in your sinus cavity increases, leading to the pain that you feel.

- *Inflammation.* Sometimes sinus pain is due to extreme swelling of the membranes against a deviated nasal septum or nerve area. Or, if you suffer sinus pain while in cold air, you may have a wide nose in which the bones don't come together. When the roof of your nose is open, cold air strikes the membranes directly, resulting in excruciating pain.

- *Referred pain.* Sometimes, what you may think is a sinus headache is really "referred" pain from the neck. This is because of the hookup of the nerves causing painful stimuli to radiate to the front of your face above your eyes.

Other Causes of Headache

Problems inside your head can cause headaches, which can be mistaken for sinus headache. A common concern you may have is that there may be a brain tumor, yet headaches are the first sign in only a third or less of brain tumors. There are usually other signs your doctor will find upon examination.

Infections, injuries to the head, inflammation of the nerves and arteries, and diseases of the eye, ear, nose, or teeth are possible causes of headaches, but they are not as common. You may be concerned that your severe headache is a sign of a stroke, but this is a very uncommon cause of chronic headaches.

Treating Headache Pain

Since each of these kinds of headaches may have treatment available, it is important to first identify the problem. Talk with your physician for advice. If the headache concerns you, let your doctor know so that this worry can be quickly eliminated with simple medical tests.

Medication

Pain Relievers.   As with most types of pain, over-the-counter analgesics such as acetaminophen, aspirin, ibuprofen, or naproxen should be tried to see if any of these alleviate the pain. If the headache persists, you may try an over-the-counter analgesic that also contains caffeine.

If over-the-counter pain relievers do not touch your headache pain, ask your doctor about a higher-dose prescription strength naproxen. The Cox-2 inhibitors (Super Aspirins) may also help give relief from pain without gastrointestinal upset. Midrin (contains a blood vessel constrictor, mild nonaddicting sedative, and acetaminophen), or Norgesic Forte (contains aspirin, caffeine, and nonaddicting muscle relaxant), are types of "combination" pills which may be useful as well.

Hormone Therapy.   In new studies, the medication Danazol was found to inhibit estrogen fluctuation and prevent migraines in 51 percent of women who were unresponsive to standard medical therapy. Other findings indicate that those who are most helped by hormonal therapy are women who suffer with premenstrual migraines. (Note: Danazol has serious side effects when taken in large amounts.)

Muscle Relaxants.   Some patients find temporary relief from headache pain with a muscle relaxant, such as tizanidine (Zanaflex) or baclofen (Lioresal). The benefit of muscle relaxants is they can be used "as needed," since they usually give rapid relief. If they provide no relief, talk to your doctor about another medication to relieve pain.

Migraine Relief.   If you are a migraine sufferer, a category of medicine called the triptans increase the level of serotonin in the brain, which reduces the dilation of blood vessels (source of the pain). When these drugs are taken at the start of a migraine, they can bring it to a halt within fifteen minutes. Sumatriptan, the first drug developed for migraine, is now joined by other triptans that are available in nasal sprays, wafers that "melt" in your mouth, or oral pill form. Sumatriptan (Imitrex) by injection works faster than anything else to halt a migraine headache, but if one triptan fails to work, another drug in that class can be tried.

Ergotamines contract smooth muscles, including those in blood vessels, reducing the dilation of the blood vessels. While ergotamines work in some patients, the side effects are not comfortable and patients with cardiovascular disease should not use these at all.

Other pain-relieving medications that diminish the frequency of migraine headaches include antiepileptic drugs (valproic acid), beta-blockers (propranolol), calcium channel blockers (verapamil), and others. A relatively new treatment approach is the use of botulinum toxins injected in the head. This therapy appears to hold some promise as a useful therapeutic tool.

If you suffer with menstrual migraines, your doctor may put you on low-dose contraceptives to try to keep the level of estrogen from falling. Falling estrogen levels trigger migraines.

Antidepressants.   Sometimes a tricyclic antidepressant, such as Elavil (amitriptyline) or Pamelor (nortriptyline) is used to address the underlying anxiety and depression problems and also help diminish the headache and decrease the pain. These drugs may also help you get restful sleep, which can also help reduce the pain. The newer selective serotonin reuptake inhibitors (SSRIs), such as Prozac (fluoxetine), Zoloft (sertraline), and Paxil (paroxetine), are also recommended by many headache experts to raise the level of serotonin in the brain associated with migraine and other headaches.

RED FLAG!

If your headaches are becoming more frequent, ask your doctor about medication-abuse headaches. If you have tension-type headaches or migraines and use pain relievers frequently, you actually may be worsening the problem. Taking analgesics, opioids, or other pain-relieving medications daily or several times a week can potentially make your headache pain less responsive to preventive medicines, causing an episodic headache to become a chronic daily headache. Try to incorporate other alternative therapies along with the medication to reduce your dependence.

Natural Cures

De-stress.   When you first feel the signs of a headache coming on, take a thirty-minute break and "chill." Lie quietly in a dark room with a warm or cool compress on your head. Close your eyes, and remove yourself from the day's stressors to see if the pain will diminish. Sometimes stopping the daily activity with a time-out helps stop headache pain.

Herbal Therapy.   Patients tell of getting headache relief from the following herbs:

- Feverfew, which appears to block a protein key to inflammation
- White willow bark, which contains salicin, a natural predecessor to aspirin
- Ginger, which has an antihistamine and anti-inflammatory action in the body

Natural Supplements.   Papaya enzyme tablets, available at most drug or natural food stores, may help headache pain if it's associated with nasal congestion or sinusitis. These tablets, held between the cheek and gums, can help to reduce inflammation associated with sinusitis, nasal inflammation, earache, or sore throat.

Hydrotherapy.   Try the following—either alone or in combination—to see which form of hydrotherapy may help reduce your pain:

- Use warm, moist cloths on the sinus area for ten to fifteen minutes, twice a day, to reduce inflammation and pain.
- Apply ice packs to the forehead (be sure to cover your skin with a towel).
- Use a combination of heat and ice, alternating every five minutes.
- Breathe steam to open nasal passages, if the headache is related to the sinus cavity.

Try Nasal Irrigation. If you have a sinus headache, use nasal irrigation—cleaning your sinuses out with mild salt water or saline solution—to remove thick mucus and stimulate natural nasal function. Saline solution is available in easy-to-use containers at most grocery and drug stores.

Exercise

Stress plays a big role in headaches, from the daily tension headache to the blinding migraines to jaw pain associated with TMJ syndrome. But exercise can literally clear your head of stress—and the subsequent pain. Getting your heart rate up also reduces stress on a chemical level.

Healing Nutrients

Migraine headaches are often caused by dietary triggers. Go through the list of foods and try to identify the ones that affect you and your headache pain, and avoid those foods that are bothersome. The National Headache Foundation lists the following foods as possible migraine or headache triggers:

- Ripened cheeses—Cheddar, Emmentaler, Stilton, Brie, and Camembert (Permissible cheeses—American, cottage, cream cheese, and Velveeta)
- Pickled or dried herring
- Chocolate
- Anything fermented, pickled, or marinated
- Sour cream (have no more than ½ cup daily)
- Nuts, peanut butter
- Sourdough bread, breads and crackers containing cheese or chocolate
- Broad beans, lima beans, fava beans, snow peas
- Foods containing monosodium glutamate (MSG)—soy sauce, meat tenderizers, seasoned salt
- Figs, raisins, papayas, avocados, red plums (no more than ½ cup daily)
- Citrus fruits (have no more than ½ cup daily)
- Bananas (have no more than ½ banana daily)
- Pizza
- Excessive amounts of tea, coffee, or cola beverages (limit to 2 cups daily)

- Sausage, bologna, pepperoni, salami, summer sausage, hot dogs
- Chicken livers, pâté
- Alcoholic beverages (If you do drink, limit yourself to two normal-size drinks.)

Mind/Body Exercises

Because of the stress-headache connection, mind/body exercises may be helpful in reducing pain. You might try the relaxation response, deep abdominal breathing, or music therapy. Aromatherapy combined with meditation often helps alleviate headache pain.

The American Headache Society and the National Headache Foundation recommend biofeedback as a way of changing your response to life's stressors, resulting in fewer headaches. During a biofeedback session, you are hooked up to electronic sensors and a monitor. The sensors project your physiological responses to various stressors on a visual monitor. After a period of time, you can learn how to exert a degree of voluntary control over certain body functions, such as heart rate.

Visualization is another excellent mind/body exercise as you imagine yourself in comforting places when you need to relax. This often helps the blood vessels to dilate, stopping the pain in its tracks.

Bodywork and Massage

The National Institutes of Health supports the use of acupuncture for headache pain when used in conjunction with a comprehensive management program. This ancient Chinese practice works with the application of hair-thin needles to specific anatomical points and is thought to release the blockages and tension that can cause pain, providing pain relief. Along the same line, acupressure, a hands-on type of acupuncture, may also help headache pain, and you can do this in the privacy of your home or office.

Some women find relief with compression, such as a soft band tightly pressed against the painful area. Others rely on regular chiropractic spinal adjustments to get relief for chronic headaches. Chiropractors and some osteopathic physicians use manipulation of joints to reduce nerve irritation and release muscle tension that is causing the headache.

High-Tech Solutions

Many chronic headache sufferers use TENS (see page 250) to get ongoing relief from pain. If you suffer with TMJ, ask your dentist about a special appliance that is worn at night to prevent you from clenching your jaw and grinding your teeth.

When to Call the Doctor

If your headache pain is extreme or progressively worsens, call your doctor for an evaluation. Or if you have headache with unending nausea, blurred vision, slurred speech, dizziness, or difficulty in sitting or standing, seek emergency treatment.

CHAPTER SIX

Fibromyalgia

Lauren, a magazine editor, constantly battled deadlines. This thirty-six-year-old mother of three said she first saw her primary care physician because she had been experiencing pain in her lower back and upper thighs when she got out of bed in the morning. Although she had been under great pressure at work, she felt unusually tired even after sleeping nine or ten hours at night. After having a physical examination and drawing blood for a laboratory test, Lauren's doctor sent her for an MRI, a noninvasive procedure that uses magnets and radio waves to produce a picture of the inside of the body area being investigated. When the test showed no abnormalities, the doctor told Lauren to take it easy and stop pushing herself. He gave her a tranquilizer to take when she felt extremely stressed, but this did not help the muscle pain and only left her feeling more tired, inattentive, and hopeless.

By the time Lauren was referred to me, she had seen four doctors about her nonspecific symptoms: the "relentless" pain in her lower back, legs, and shoulders; along with chronic headaches, irritable bowels, and periodic feelings of high anxiety. To maintain enough energy to keep her job at the magazine, Lauren went to bed immediately after dinner each night while her husband managed the family. She said her marriage was suffering, as her husband thought the pain and fatigue were "in her head," and she did not know how long she could continue working as an editor as she could not concentrate much of the time.

After reviewing her previous tests and ruling out other more serious diseases, I explained to Lauren that she had fibromyalgia syndrome, a commonly misdiagnosed and misunderstood syndrome and *the* most common arthritis-related illness next to osteoarthritis. With fibromyalgia the constant pain and suffering are intertwined with ongoing feelings of fatigue, which lead to unending depression and social isolation. I recommended medications to help ease the pain and to promote sounder sleep at night. Lauren then began the 8-step program in part 3 of this book, focusing on changing her diet, increasing daily stretching and resistance exercises, and using the mind/body exercises to help her cope with daily stressors.

In my practice, I treat many women like Lauren, who have gone from doctor to doctor seeking answers for their deep muscle pain and other nonspecific symptoms. Nonetheless, whether fibromyalgia syndrome or another problem is causing the pain, I know these women have other burdens along with the symptoms they feel, and usually caring for others comes before important self-care. These women are the ones who care for the babies, pick up children from school, carpool their children to extracurricular activities, review homework, prepare meals for the family, do the household chores, and also work full-time jobs outside the home. The painful and relentless symptoms of fibromyalgia (or other pain problems), combined with the ongoing caregiving tasks, put enormous physical and psychological strains on women, and can disrupt marital intimacy and family relationships and lead to loss of work hours, reduced income, and even job loss.

What Is Fibromyalgia Syndrome?

Fibromyalgia syndrome (FMS) is a complex rheumatic-type disorder characterized by widespread pain, decreased pain threshold or tender points, and incapacitating fatigue. These symptoms affect more than 10 million Americans, mostly women between twenty-five and sixty. In fact, women are ten times more likely to get this disease than men. While there is no specific laboratory test or abnormal X ray finding to diagnosis fibromyalgia, the symptoms of the disease can be successfully treated *once a proper diagnosis is made by your physician.*

What You Might Feel: Signs and Symptoms

Fibromyalgia causes you to literally ache all over. You may have symptoms of crippling fatigue, specific "tender points" on the body that are painful to touch, swelling, disturbances in deep-level or restful sleep, and mood disturbances or depression. Your muscles may feel as if they have been overworked or pulled without exercising or other cause. Sometimes your muscles twitch, burn, or have deep stabbing pain. Some women have pain and achiness around the joints in the neck, shoulder, back, and hips, making it difficult to sleep or exercise. Other symptoms you might feel include:

- Fatigue upon arising
- Difficulty maintaining sleep or light sleep
- Stiffness
- Hypersensitivity to cold and/or heat
- Abdominal pain
- Chronic headaches
- Numbness or tingling in the fingers and feet
- Irritable bowel syndrome
- Incontinence
- Anxiety and depression
- Inability to concentrate (called "fibro fog")
- Poor circulation in hands and feet (Raynaud's phenomenon)
- Restless legs syndrome
- Dryness in mouth, nose, and eyes
- Painful menstrual cramps

Because fibromyalgia can cause signs and feelings similar to osteoarthritis, bursitis, and tendinitis, some experts include it in this group of arthritis and related disorders. But unlike the bursitis or tendinitis that is localized to a single area, the pain and stiffness of fibromyalgia are very widespread.

FIBROMYALGIA TRIGGERS

- Fatigue
- Changes in weather (cold or humidity)
- Physical exhaustion
- Lack of sleep or restless sleep

- Sedentary lifestyle
- Anxiety and depression

What Causes Fibromyalgia?

Probably one of the toughest things I have to do as a pain specialist is to tell a woman I really don't know what caused her problem. At this time, the causes of fibromyalgia are virtually unknown. Investigators have been looking at hormonal disturbances and chemical imbalances that affect nerve signaling. While just speculation right now, it may be that lower levels of serotonin in the blood leads to lowered pain thresholds. (Serotonin, a neurotransmitter in the brain, is associated with a calming, anxiety-reducing reaction.) This may be caused by the reduced effectiveness of the body's natural endorphin painkillers, discussed on page 180, and the increased presence of "substance P," which increases pain perception. The situation is extremely complex and may be more related to a maldistribution of serotonin. Increased serotonin in some areas may facilitate pain, and medications which block serotonin may actually help pain and fibromyalgia. Still, these theories are merely speculative.

Some researchers theorize that stress and poor physical conditioning are both major factors in the cause of fibromyalgia. Or that muscle microtrauma (tiny amounts of damage) leads to calcium leakage, which increases muscle contraction, further reducing the oxygen supply. This process appears to be linked with a reduction in the muscle's ability to produce energy, causing it to fatigue and to be unable to pump the excess calcium out of the cells.

Most of my FMS patients experience nonrestorative sleep, such as insomnia or light and unrefreshing sleep. It may be that disordered sleep leads to the lower levels of serotonin, resulting in increased pain sensitivity. Researchers have demonstrated what amounts to lower pain threshold induced by sleep deprivation in healthy women, which is also associated with an abnormal brain wave pattern.

Other researchers believe that because fibromyalgia is accompanied by low-grade depression, there may be a link between the two illnesses. Another theory states that fibromyalgia is caused by biochemical changes in the body and may be related to hormonal changes or menopause. Still other studies reveal that fibromyalgia may result from sudden trauma to the central nervous system.

Like other rheumatic diseases, fibromyalgia could be the result of a genetic tendency, passed from mother to daughter. When a woman with this tendency is exposed to certain emotional or physical stressors (like a traumatic crisis or a serious illness), there is a change in her body's response to stress. Scientists theorize that one of these body changes is a low level of the hormone CRH (corticotropin-releasing hormone), resulting in higher sensitivity to pain and more fatigue, including the fatigue experienced after exercise. This hypersensitivity to pain may in part be from low levels of serotonin. Lower levels of serotonin cause a lower pain threshold and disordered sleep. The end result may be the chronic widespread pain of fibromyalgia. Some studies show that women have approximately seven times less serotonin in the brain, which may explain why FMS is more prevalent in women than in men. Abnormal transport of serum tryptophan (a precursor for serotonin) has also been described in clinical findings.

There is simply no single theory that explains who is at risk for fibromyalgia. Whatever the cause, the unending pain and interrupted sleep are guaranteed to increase the fatigue and depression you feel, leading to increased anxiety, reduced activity, and greater pain. Disordered sleep can reduce your energy levels, and if continued over time, can lead to a decrease in repair to damaged tissues. Once your doctor makes a proper diagnosis, effective treatment can be started to manage the symptoms before you lose quality of life.

ARE YOU AT RISK?

While researchers have identified some common risk factors for fibromyalgia, there are still many patients with the disease who have none of these traits or markers at all. Also, some women have fibromyalgia without any other underlying disease, while others have fibromyalgia along with diseases such as osteoarthritis, rheumatoid arthritis, or systemic lupus erythematosus. Possible risk factors for fibromyalgia include:

- Gender (usually female)
- Genetic disposition (may be inherited)
- Poor physical conditioning
- Personality (perfectionist)
- Trauma to the central nervous system (after an injury, accident, illness, or emotional stress)

- Depression
- Surgery
- Menopause (loss of estrogen)

How Is Fibromyalgia Diagnosed?

There is no laboratory test or X ray that can diagnose fibromyalgia, so talking to your doctor and describing how you feel is usually the most important tool for arriving at the correct clinical diagnosis. A comprehensive physical examination and the patient's medical history, as well as a *diagnosis of exclusion* (ruling out other diagnoses that can be causing similar symptoms) is critical. I also use a *diagnosis of inclusion*—making sure the woman's symptoms satisfy the diagnostic criteria outlined by the American College of Rheumatology. These criteria include widespread pain (pain in the right and left sides of the body, above and below the waist, involving the chest, neck, mid or lower back) which persists for at least three months, and pain evoked by a specific pressure in at least eleven of eighteen specific anatomic sites.

Your doctor will run some specific blood tests, described in Step 2, such as a complete blood count (CBC). Tests of other chemicals, such as glucose, that can create problems similar to fibromyalgia will be done, as well as thyroid tests. An underactive thyroid (hypothyroidism), caused by reduced hormone production by the thyroid gland, can cause problems similar to fibromyalgia with the fatigue, muscle aches, weakness, and depression.

Other laboratory tests may include tests for Lyme disease, antinuclear antibodies (ANA), rheumatoid factor (RF), erythrocyte sedimentation rate (ESR), prolactin level and calcium level (parathyroid abnormalities).

Although fibromyalgia does not cause changes that show up on X rays, your doctor may still want to rule out more serious causes of pain by taking routine X rays or even ordering an MRI.

Treating Fibromyalgia Syndrome

There is no known cure for fibromyalgia, but I find great success using a multifaceted treatment program that includes a combination of medications, muscle therapy, aerobic conditioning, and behavioral techniques (all discussed in the 8-step program to end pain).

Many women with fibromyalgia are able to greatly reduce their pain, anxiety, depression, and fatigue, and increase healing sleep, by undertaking this treatment program.

Medications

Pharmacologic treatment rarely eliminates all the deep muscle or joint pain or normalizes other symptoms you may feel, such as fatigue or sleep. Nevertheless, medications can help you to better manage your pain. I recommend medications such as antidepressants (amitriptyline, or Elavil), muscle relaxants (cyclobenzaprine, or Flexeril), and analgesics (tramadol, or Ultram), explained in Step 2. Although traditionally nonsteroidal anti-inflammatory drugs (NSAIDs) have not been especially helpful for FMS patients, they are often useful to try if you have a wide spectrum of musculoskeletal complaints. Many find the new Cox-2 inhibitors work well to ease pain and reduce inflammation without causing gastrointestinal distress. Tizanidine (Zanaflex) is a medication that may have great benefit for FMS patients. This medication helps with sleep, pain, and muscle spasms and restless leg movements, as well as diminishes the amount of substance P in the cerebrospinal fluid.

Additional treatment strategies that may be useful for specific areas of pain include patches of prescription lidocaine (a local anesthetic similar to novocaine), capsaicin (from hot chili peppers), or a salve "cocktail" of multiple pain-relieving ingredients (prescription), which are generally prepared by an experienced compounding pharmacist.

Natural Cures

Dietary Supplements.   Fibromyalgia's nonspecific pain lends itself to various natural therapies. To ease the anxiety and depression that accompanies FMS, some patients have found SAM-e, 5-HTP, kava, and St. John's wort to be effective (do not take these with other antidepressants). Valerian or melatonin may help you fall asleep more easily and sleep through the night without interruption. For pain, patients with fibromyalgia have successfully tried the herbs feverfew, white willow, and devil's claw, as well as fish oil (EPA), borage seed oil, and evening primrose oil—all natural supplements discussed in Step 5.

Studies on Super Malic, a supplement that contains malic acid (200 mg) and magnesium (50 mg) show that it may help to ease the overall pain of fibromyalgia patients.

Hydrotherapy.   Many of my patients also find long-lasting relief with hydrotherapy, either hot or cold modalities. In fact, balneotherapy, or the use of hot baths or spas to alleviate pain, is a centuries-old therapy that helps to increase muscle relaxation, boost blood supply to the site, and relieve rigidity and spasms in the muscles of patients with fibromyalgia.

Salves and Liniments.   If heat is comforting over a painful body area, then Kwan Loong Oil (nonprescription) may also help in alleviating pain. This "super Ben Gay–type" preparation is often available stores that sell Asian products.

Exercise

If your fibromyalgia leaves you feeling "stressed out" frequently, exercise can help desensitize your body to stress. A study published in February 2002 in *Arthritis Care and Research* confirms that a combination of cardiovasvular exercise and strength training helps women with fibromyalgia increase their strength and endurance, and reduce their fatigue, pain, stiffness, and depression. Some simple ways to incorporate these two types of exercise are suggested in Step 4.

Healing Nutrients

As with any chronic disease, the foods you eat play a key role in healing and wellness, and nutrients are especially important for staying well. Information presented in 2001 at the American College of Nutrition suggests that eliminating some foods may help those with fibromyalgia feel less pain and fatigue. In the study, women with FMS eliminated from their diet such common foods as corn, wheat, dairy, citrus, soy, and nuts. After two weeks without eating any of the trigger foods, almost half of the fibromyalgia patients claimed a significant reduction of pain. About 76 percent said there was a reduction in symptoms such as headache, fatigue, bloating, heartburn, and breathing difficulties. Patients then slowly added back the offending foods to see which ones triggered FMS symptoms. When they noticed symptoms, such as increased pain or headache, they were instructed to avoid that food. The elimination diet is explained in Step 5, so you can see if this may help you find a link between the food you eat and your fibromyalgia symptoms.

Antioxidants Give Cell Protection.   Antioxidants, essential nutrients that help protect your body against life's stressors, are found in food sources rich in beta-carotene and vitamins C and E. Antioxidants are thought to play a role in the body's cell-protection system by neutralizing highly reactive and unstable molecules, called free radicals, produced by the body. In research, free radicals have been shown to disrupt and tear apart vital cell structures like cell membranes. Antioxidants have been shown to tie up these free radicals and take away their destructive power—perhaps reducing the risk of a number of chronic diseases and even slowing the aging process. Eating to heal FMS requires a diet rich in antioxidants.

Some researchers think that antioxidants might help prevent damage in some types of arthritis and boost immune function when a system is under stress.

Protein Builds Body Tissue and Fights Infection.   Protein is also important to build and repair body tissue and fight infection. Too little protein in the diet may lead to symptoms of fatigue, weakness, apathy, and poor immunity. Average-size adult women need 45–55 grams of protein a day, and more protein if there is fever or infection.

One ounce of meat, chicken, cheese, or fish provides 7 grams of protein; one cup of milk, 8 grams. Therefore, 5–6 ounces of meat per day and 2 cups of milk provide adequate protein for most adults. You can also substitute vegetable proteins such as soy products or lentils to meet your daily requirement.

Carbohydrates Boost Serotonin.   Nutritional factors, including certain carbohydrate foods, may also have a positive effect on serotonin. In Step 5, I explain how to use these foods to boost serotonin and increase calmness.

Add Zinc.   Zinc has tremendous antioxidant effects and is vital to your body's resistance to infection and for tissue repair. Many illnesses, including kidney disease and long-term infection, are associated with zinc deficiency. If you are taking medication, it may interfere with zinc absorption in the intestines and cause a zinc deficiency. To improve immune function, eat foods high in zinc, including seafood, eggs, meats, whole grains, wheat germ, nuts, and seeds. Avoid coffee, tea, and diuretics containing tannins—substances that contract tissues and may hinder zinc absorption.

Mind/Body Exercises

Support groups are of particular benefit to those with fibromyalgia. Within these groups, you can share how FMS affects your life: what you feel, the frustrations you face, the therapies that are helpful, and how the illness impacts your relationships and your work. Other mind/body modalities that may be useful include relaxation techniques, guided imagery, hypnotherapy, biofeedback, and meditation, among others. Psychotherapy and cognitive behavioral techniques, such as positive self-talks and autogenic therapy, a series of simple body awareness exercises that help switch the body from the "fight or flight" system into relaxation mode, also have potential value and may help you gain effective coping skills.

Disturbed sleep and the resulting exhaustion you feel causes reduced physical fitness and the establishment of a vicious cycle of inactivity and sleep disturbance with physical and mood-related symptoms. Because patients with fibromyalgia have a specific type of disordered sleep, including insomnia, that may lead to the feelings of achiness and fatigue, relaxation therapies may help in reducing high levels of arousal before bedtime and allowing for more restful sleep. The use of a special mattress pad made from sheep's wool may help. The mattress is called "Cuddle Ewe" and can be found at www.ImmuneSupport.com.

Bodywork and Massage

Bodywork, massage, and other hands-on therapies give great relief to many women with fibromyalgia as muscle tension is relieved. Deep tissue massage may help release muscle tension that increases pain.

High-Tech Solutions

In some women, more high-tech solutions are necessary to alleviate deep muscle pain. Ask your doctor about galvanic ultrasound and TENS, described in Step 8. If there is significant muscle tightness without great relief from a steroid injection, other injections such as botulinum toxins around the spine may help to alleviate the severe, chronic pain.

When to Call the Doctor

It's important to know that some internal organ problems can cause chronic pain that may mimic the overall aching and throbbing muscle pain of fibromyalgia. If the pain is caused by kidney disease, stomach disease, or other internal organ abnormality, treating the problem will resolve the pain. Cancer and other serious diseases can mimic the symptoms of fatigue and weakness. In many cases, early treatment can essentially eliminate the problem and the symptoms. That's why an accurate diagnosis is so important. After you have been diagnosed with fibromyalgia, should any of the symptoms worsen with prescribed treatment or alternative therapies, call your doctor. You may need a different medication or medical therapy, or you may have a new or coexisting problem that needs to be diagnosed and resolved.

CHAPTER SEVEN

Arthritis

While many view arthritis as a disease of the elderly, this is entirely inaccurate. Three out of five arthritis patients are under the age of sixty-five. Osteoarthritis, a progressive deterioration in the cartilage of certain joints, including the knee and vertebrae, can result from overuse of joints or is often a consequence of demanding sports, obesity, or aging. Osteoarthritis in the hands is often inherited and usually happens in younger women. If you were an athlete or dancer in high school or college and wonder why your knee or hip aches when you climb out of bed in the morning, ask your doctor about osteoarthritis—for it may strike early in life if you were athletic or suffered an injury. No matter when or where arthritis strikes, this painful condition is considered to be one of the most debilitating diseases of aging, and rates of the disorder are expected to rise as life expectancy increases.

Mindy was forty-nine when she was diagnosed with osteoarthritis in the shoulder. An avid tennis player in her twenties and thirties, she could barely swing a racket, much less brush her hair, when I first treated her. An elementary school teacher, she found it difficult even to pick up the box of take-home papers to grade, as any lifting triggered intense pain. She had tried nonsteroid anti-inflammatory drugs (NSAIDs) but with a history of stomach problems, she couldn't take these medications without feeling indigestion and nausea. Though she thought she'd just learn to live with the pain, this changed dramatically when her new granddaughter was born. When Mindy could not hold the baby, she sought new treatment to end her discomfort and to regain her active life.

Mindy started taking one of the new Cox-2 inhibitors (Super Aspirin) that was formulated specifically for those with osteoarthritis. She also began regular applications of moist heat, along with stretching exercises to strengthen the muscles that support the shoulder joint. In less than three weeks of self-care, Mindy was virtually pain-free. Not only did the osteoarthritis pain subside, but her range of motion and strength greatly improved. At her last visit, she said she rejoined her tennis team and babysits on the weekends for her granddaughter when she doesn't have a tournament.

Elizabeth's story is typical of many middle-aged women with osteoarthritis who think that if they ignore the pain, it will go away. Arthritis pain does *not* go away! This forty-three-year-old attorney suffered with severe pain in her knees for years. The pain had started in her twenties when she was dancing with a local ballet company while attending law school. Not wanting to admit there was a more serious problem, Elizabeth said she took up to ten nonsteroid anti-inflammatory pills a day to get relief—until she felt a gnawing, burning pain in her stomach. When Elizabeth could not put weight on her leg as she stepped off the subway, she realized she needed a more effective treatment.

After a series of tests, Elizabeth was diagnosed with osteoarthritis. I recommended that she take over-the-counter acetaminophen (Tylenol) to help ease the pain, and also the natural supplement glucosamine, which seems to have the same analgesic effect as nonsteroid anti-inflammatory drugs. Elizabeth began a regular program of moist heat, twice daily, to help with pain and stiffness and started swimming laps several times each week at the local "Y" to help build strength and lose weight.

In less than two weeks, Elizabeth noticed a great reduction in pain, and she was able to start walking during her lunch hour to increase her amount of exercise, which is known to improve strength and overall function of the joint. Within three months, Elizabeth had lost eleven pounds and reported having no knee pain as long as she stayed with the program. She was thrilled with the relief she felt and was enjoying her normal activities at home and at work without any pain or limitation.

Osteoarthritis

Of the more than 100 types of arthritis, osteoarthritis (OA), the "wear-and-tear" arthritis, is the most common, affecting more than 15 million women. While women account for about 65 percent of all arthritis cases, they account for 74 percent of osteoarthritis cases. The risk of getting osteoarthritis increases with age, especially after age forty.

Osteoarthritis is most common in weight-bearing joints—the knees, hips, feet, and spine—and often comes on gradually over months or years. Except for the intense pain in the affected joint, you usually do not feel sick, and there is no unusual fatigue or tiredness as with the more serious inflammatory types of arthritis, such as rheumatoid.

What You Might Feel: Signs and Symptoms

In osteoarthritis, you may feel fine except for the painful joint involved. There may be a few minutes of stiffness on arising in the morning, and there may be some stiffness after sitting for a short period of time. However, these symptoms are usually not as severe as with inflammatory types of arthritis such as rheumatoid.

SYMPTOMS OF OSTEOARTHRITIS INCLUDE:

- Deep, aching pain in joint
- Swelling of joint
- Joint may be warm to touch
- Morning stiffness
- Stiffness after resting
- Fatigue
- Pain when walking
- Difficulty gripping objects
- Difficulty dressing or combing hair
- Difficulty sitting or bending over

What Causes Osteoarthritis?

As you get older, or if you have previous injuries to your joints, there may be minor damage to the cartilage that cannot be completely repaired. Gradually, as more and more damage happens, the cartilage begins to wear away or it doesn't work as well to cushion your joint. As the cartilage becomes worn, the smoothness of cartilage cushioning the joint is lost. This can cause pain when the joint is moved. Along with the pain, sometimes you may hear a grating sound when the roughened cartilage on the surface of the bones rubs together.

ARE YOU AT RISK?

Risk Factors for Osteoarthritis

- Age (risk increases with age)
- Injury
- Heavy, constant joint use
- Athletics (wear and tear and injuries)
- Overweight
- Knee surgery
- Abnormal joint positions
- Changing forces (putting weight on one knee or hip)
- Joint injury by other types of arthritis
- Gender (osteoarthritis is more common in women)
- Lack of exercise (weak muscles giving no support to aging joints)

How Is Osteoarthritis Diagnosed?

Blood tests can help eliminate other more serious inflammatory types of arthritis and other medical problems, while a sample of the joint fluid from the knee can also show typical changes of osteoarthritis. Usually by the time a patient gets treatment, changes are visible on an X ray of the joint. A narrowing of the cartilage may show on the X ray, but no destruction as with rheumatoid arthritis.

Rheumatoid Arthritis

Inflammatory types of arthritis occur when your immune system goes haywire and attacks the linings of your joints. Almost any joint can be involved, and the causes of only a few types are known.

Although there are many types of inflammatory arthritis, rheumatoid arthritis is the most common and is caused by the body's immune response. With rheumatoid, joint pain, swelling, and stiffness can be severe and even crippling. In about 20 percent of those with rheumatoid arthritis, lumps—called *rheumatoid nodules*—may develop over joint areas that receive pressure, such as knuckles of the hand, elbows, or heels.

What You Might Feel: Signs and Symptoms

Rheumatoid arthritis acts differently than osteoarthritis. The symptoms usually come on gradually. However, in some cases, the symptoms start suddenly and are much more severe than those of osteoarthritis. For instance, twenty-two-year-old Laura, a college student, woke up one day feeling feverish and with both knees stiff and swollen—the first sign she had that something was amiss in her body. Up until that morning, she had felt no pain at all. With rheumatoid arthritis, you may feel pain and stiffness and experience swelling in the hands, wrists, elbows, shoulders, knees, ankles, feet, jaws, or neck.

Sometimes this pain occurs in one body part, but it usually occurs in combinations, such as in the hands, knees, and feet. In rheumatoid arthritis, the joints tend to be involved in a symmetrical pattern. That is, if the knuckles on the left hand are inflamed, the knuckles on the right hand will also be inflamed. After a period of time, more of your joints may gradually become involved with pain and swelling and may feel warm to the touch. The joint swelling is constant and interferes with the very activities that allow us to function in our daily lives—opening a jar, driving, working, and walking.

Stiffness on arising in the morning, which may have begin as a temporary nuisance, can soon last for hours or even most of the day. You will feel debilitating fatigue that is often quite severe. You may lose weight although your eating habits have not changed. Fever, rash, and even internal organ involvement of the heart or lungs can occur with rheumatoid arthritis when the immune system spills over from the joints to other areas of the body. The exact causes of rashes and heart and lung involvement are not known.

What Causes Rheumatoid Arthritis?

With rheumatoid arthritis, although the precise cause is unknown, some of your body's cells may recognize a protein as a foreign intruder. (The exact proteins involved in rheumatoid arthritis has not yet been discovered.) Certain cells called lymphocytes are stimulated to react to this protein. The reaction causes the release of chemicals called cytokines, which are messengers that then trigger more inflammation and destruction from other cells. This battle between the body's chemicals occurs mainly in the joints, but can spill over to other areas of the body.

There are many cytokines, but the most important so far in causing inflammation are tumor necrosis factor (TNF) and interlukin-1. These are thought to trigger many of the other enzymes in rheumatoid arthritis. Researchers believe that if TNF and interlukin-1 are blocked, many of the reactions that damage joints could be improved, and many of the other symptoms of arthritis, such as fatigue, may be helped.

WHO'S AT RISK?

Rheumatoid arthritis is the most common type of inflammatory arthritis, with more than ten million Americans affected. Like osteoarthritis, this inflammatory arthritis is more common in women. More than 70 percent of all rheumatoid arthritis cases affect women (about 1.5 million), and it's usually diagnosed between ages twenty and fifty.

How Is Rheumatoid Arthritis Diagnosed?

Your doctor will make the diagnosis of rheumatoid arthritis after doing a thorough physical examination, along with X rays and certain blood tests, such as the rheumatoid factor. The rheumatoid factor, an indicator of inflammation, is positive in 70 to 80 percent of those with rheumatoid arthritis. Keep in mind that the rheumatoid factor is not specific for rheumatoid arthritis—meaning you can have this without having rheumatoid arthritis—but it does give your doctor useful information when combined with other signs and symptoms such as pain, swelling, and stiffness.

While there are many diagnostic tools, X rays are most useful in helping your doctor detect rheumatoid arthritis in its early stages, when it is very treatable. Images taken of the hands, wrists, and feet are the most useful to show early changes, as the disease attacks these areas first. X rays show the first permanent changes in joints and can alert your doctor to start the latest and most effective treatments early in the disease—when treatment is most beneficial and damage is least. The right treatments can actually delay or stop the progress of the bone damage and destruction and can help prevent deformity in the end.

Systemic Lupus Erythematosus (SLE or Lupus)

Systemic lupus erythematosus (SLE or lupus) is another inflammatory type of arthritis and is more common in women. With SLE there is inflammation in the blood vessels that can cause serious damage to many organs. Fever, rash, heart disease, seizures, blood disorders, and many other life-threatening complications can happen.

What You Might Feel: Signs and Symptoms

With SLE, you will feel pain in many joints, fatigue, and stiffness in the morning. Rashes are common, including the "butterfly rash" across the cheeks in about 15 to 20 percent of cases. There may be an unusual sensitivity to sunlight that causes a rash and other illness. Hair loss, discoloration of the fingers or toes when exposed to cold (Raynaud's phenomenon), and other internal organ damage can occur. Half of those with SLE also have kidney disease. Coexisting blood disorders can cause anemia and blood clots. Chest pain from heart and lung inflammation can happen, and seizures or strokes can occur.

What Causes Lupus?

While the cause of SLE is not known, it appears that the body reacts to certain proteins, which it recognizes as foreign. This reaction causes certain cells to create inflammation through cytokines, which are released. The cytokines give "messages" to cause arthritis in the joints. Yet, with SLE, the inflammation is not only in joints, but also commonly in many internal organs, especially the kidneys.

WHO'S AT RISK?

SLE is most common in younger women, ages twenty to forty, and is more common in African American women. More than 90 percent of systemic lupus erythematosus cases in the United States are women.

How Is Lupus Diagnosed?

Blood tests, especially the antinuclear antibody test (ANA), can help in diagnosing SLE. About 95 percent of active cases of SLE have a positive ANA blood test, although everyone with a positive test does not necessarily have SLE. Antinuclear antibodies are found in patients whose immune system is prone to cause inflammation against their own body tissues. Once your doctor evaluates the clinical findings and blood tests, he or she can decide if your symptoms suggest SLE and start you on the proper treatment.

WHAT IS LYME DISEASE?

Lyme disease (Lyme arthritis) is a recently discovered type of infectious arthritis caused by the Borrelia burgdorferi organism. It is most common in spring and summer months when field mice and deer carry this organism and pass it onto ticks. The ticks bite humans, resulting in a host of flulike symptoms, such as headache, joint and muscle pain, fever, chills, sore throat, stiff neck, and fatigue. You may not even realize you were bitten by a tick when the symptoms hit. Sometimes a transient faint but characteristic rash called erythema chronica migrans is present early on.

As Lyme disease progresses, the nerves become involved, and headaches and weakness are common. Bell's palsy (facial weakness) can occur at this point, and heart disease occurs in approximately 10 percent of those infected. After a period of several years, some people with Lyme disease develop chronic arthritis pain, stiffness, and swelling in the joints. Your doctor can make a diagnosis based on symptoms, history, and blood test results.

Carpal Tunnel Syndrome

Carpal tunnel syndrome (CTS) is a condition in which the median nerve, which travels down the arm into the hand, becomes compressed as it passes through a narrow path or tunnel at the wrist.

What You Might Feel: Signs and Symptoms

The symptoms of CTS include pain, tingling, or numbness in the thumb and next three fingers with the exception of the little finger. You may also feel swelling in your fingers. Sometimes pain may travel from the hand up the arm, possibly to the elbow or occasionally even to the shoulder.

The pain, numbness, and tingling usually worsen at night and while driving, holding the telephone, or maneuvering a computer mouse. Some claim the symptoms increase when the hand is warm and decrease when it is cool. You may even wake up with your hand or hands asleep and have to shake it to try to regain feeling.

As CTS progresses, your hand may become noticeably weaker, so that daily activities such as opening a jar or grasping your hairbrush may be difficult. You may drop items easily and think you're just plain clumsy when, in fact, the CTS has weakened your grip.

What Causes Carpal Tunnel Syndrome?

Overuse of the hands can cause the tissues in the area to swell, which causes compression of the median nerve. CTS can occur at any age but occurs more frequently without cause in those age fifty and up. It affects two million Americans at a cost to business of $20 billion annually, and is also reported 1.7 times more often by working women than men. More women than men also experience musculo-skeletal injuries to the hand, wrist, arm, and shoulder caused by child care responsibilities requiring lifting and bending. Younger people usually get CTS because of an injury or repetitive strain on the wrist, such as by frequent computer use.

Sometimes CTS happens because of diabetes or pregnancy, especially when someone has swelling in the hands. This swelling causes pressure on the median nerve as it travels through the bones in the wrist, which form the carpal tunnel. When the swelling improves, the symptoms may also improve.

How Is CTS Diagnosed?

Your doctor can diagnose CTS after a complete physical examination and review of your medical history. He will notice the type of pain you have and the specific places on your hand. Tests, including an electrical nerve conduction test, may be helpful in obtaining an accurate diagnosis. With CTS, X rays and blood tests are usually normal.

WHAT IS BURSITIS?

Bursitis is inflammation of one of the sacs around tendons or muscles that allow them to have smoother movements. With bursitis, you will have pain any time your muscles or tendons move—when there is movement of the joint or even pressure on the joint. The pain can be mild or severe and may last for days, weeks, or months. This can happen around the shoulders, hips, knees, elbows or buttocks. Repetitive movements, such as throwing, painting, or yard work, can frequently trigger an attack of bursitis, especially if the activity is not done regularly.

There are many different causes of bursitis, but the most common type is caused by wear-and-tear changes and repetitive movements of the muscles and tendons as they slide through the bursa sac.

WHAT IS TENDINITIS?

Tendinitis is inflammation of one of the tendons that attaches a muscle to a bone. This can cause severe pain, especially when the muscle is used. One of the most common types of tendinitis occurs at the elbow, where it is called "tennis elbow," because the movements in tennis can trigger an attack. Other common sites are the shoulder (rotator cuff tendinitis or impingement syndrome), wrist and thumb (de Quervain's disease), knee (jumper's knee), and ankle (Achilles tendinitis).

Treating Arthritis and Other Aches and Pains

Medications

Medications to Relieve Pain.   Pain relief for arthritis usually falls into two categories: (1) *Nonsteroidal anti-inflammatory drugs (NSAIDs)*, including over-the-counter aspirin, ibuprofen, ketoprofen, and naproxen sodium, which relieve pain and reduce inflammation but may cause gastrointestinal upset; and (2) *Acetaminophen*, a powerful pain reliever which, if taken over a long period of time or in large doses, can cause liver damage.

While the newer Cox-2 inhibitors (Super Aspirin) are not stronger than NSAIDs, they can eliminate pain and inflammation without the gastrointestinal side effects. In many cases, patients who take NSAIDs have to stop because of chronic indigestion or even ulcers, even though they were getting excellent relief of arthritis pain. Super Aspirins allow arthritis patients to stay on the drugs longer, so they can get optimum pain relief and become active again.

Ultracet, a short-term medication, when taken with a nonsteroid anti-inflammatory drug, has been found to give more pain relief than the NSAID taken alone. This relief is felt within a few hours and can help osteoarthritis patients who have a flare-up and need a medication boost. Calming the flare-ups is the first step in regaining control of your pain and your life. In Step 2, I introduce other medications being developed for pain, such as the sodium channel blockers, as well as medications containing chemicals from plants like chili peppers, that reduce inflammation in arthritis.

Medications for Inflammatory Types of Arthritis.　New cases of rheumatoid arthritis are treated aggressively, because damage can happen quickly without treatment to slow the disease. Your doctor may use low-dose prednisone, along with disease–modifying antirheumatic drugs, to slow down damage. To treat pain, your doctor may give you a Cox-2 inhibitor or traditional NSAID, along with your current medication. There is also a group of rheumatoid arthritis medicines described in Step 2 that take longer to work but may suppress your arthritis at a more basic level. These new breakthrough medicines can give great relief with very few side effects and work by stopping the arthritis at an earlier stage than NSAIDs.

These new rheumatoid arthritis medicines—such as Minocycline, Kineret, and Cytoxan, among others—may take one to three months to show effectiveness, but they offer 70 to 80 percent chance of improvement and increase the chance of complete control of your arthritis.

Your doctor or arthritis specialist will help you choose which of the slow-acting medicines to try first. Try to be patient and allow the total treatment of moist heat, exercises, medication, and diet, along with complementary treatments, to stop your arthritis pain.

Injections.　Hyalgan, Synvisc, and Orthovisc [sodium hyaluronate] (hyaluronic acid) are treatments for arthritis that are given by injection directly into the joint. Such injections or the use of corticosteroids are sometimes used to relieve the inflammation and pain of carpal tunnel syndrome and some types of bursitis and tendinitis. To get optimum pain relief, continue with medication, if your doctor has prescribed it, as well as the moist heat or ice, exercise, and alternative therapies of choice.

Narcotics.　During arthritis flares or when the disease has not been treated correctly, opioid (narcotic) painkillers are often used to give relief from pain.

Antibiotics for Infectious Arthritis. For all stages of Lyme disease, as well as for some other types of infectious arthritis, antibiotics are the standard form of treatment. Especially if given in the early stages, antibiotics such as penicillin or tetracycline work well. However, if there are heart problems or arthritis symptoms, higher doses of penicillin or other antibiotics are necessary.

Natural Cures

Hydrotherapy. No matter which type of arthritis you have, applications of heat or ice can help decrease pain and inflammation and increase mobility in your joints. Start with moist heat, and use this for fifteen minutes. If this does not give ample relief, use an ice pack (wrapped in a towel to protect your skin from damage), and leave it on the inflamed joint or muscle. Find the treatment that works best for you, then continue to use it at least twice daily for optimal relief.

Glucosamine Helps Repair Cartilage. The natural over-the-counter supplement glucosamine works for many women in alleviating the pain and stiffness of arthritis. In the body, glucosamine is a naturally occurring amino sugar found in human joints and connective tissues. The body uses it for cartilage development and repair. You may find that the liquid form of glucosamine is the most effective.

Dietary Supplements. Some women find pain relief with SAM-e, which is thought to have mild anti-inflammatory, pain-relieving, and tissue-healing properties. This over-the-counter supplement is a stabilized, synthetic form of S-adenosylmethionine (SAM), which is a chemical produced naturally in all animals.

Many other herbal therapies, discussed in Step 3, may give relief to arthritis pain including boswellia, white willow bark, and feverfew.

Rubs and Salves. Many of my patients find excellent relief with rubs and salves, including over-the-counter products such as Aspercreme and Ben-Gay. One particularly beneficial product is cayenne, found in Zostrix, Capzasin P, and Dolorac. Cayenne contains a substance known as capsaicin—a common remedy for arthritis pain when rubbed on the skin. Capsaicin relieves pain by acting on the sensory nerves and giving a counterirritant effect (something that causes irritation to a tissue to which it is applied, distracting from the original irritation—joint pain).

Exercise

Exercise helps improve the flexibility of your arthritic joints and keeps them from becoming stiff and immovable. It also helps improve the strength of the muscles that support your joints. When your joints have strong muscles supporting them, they are likely to have less inflammation, less pain, and less stiffness. And the stronger you are, the less likely you are to fall, which can be devastating for someone with painful arthritis.

The type of exercise you choose should greatly depend on the type and location of your arthritis. For example, swimming is excellent for osteoarthritis in the hips and knees as it strengthens the muscles around the joints while placing little stress on the joints. If you have rheumatoid arthritis, you may also find that swimming or water exercises help reduce pain all over your body and keep you flexible. Talk to your doctor or a physical therapist to find specific exercises that will help boost muscle strength and keep your joints moving in full range of motion.

Ancient Disciplines.   Both yoga and tai chi are proven to ease stress and increase relaxation and an awareness of the body. In a study presented in December 2001 at the annual meeting of the American College of Rheumatology, researchers working with osteoarthritis patients concluded that tai chi helps to improve strength, balance, and flexibility through gentle movements.

The Pilates Method.   The Pilates method is another excellent exercise that gives relief for those with arthritis. Pilates is a series of movements that you do on special equipment under supervision of a professional instructor. This method focuses on flexibility and works to "lengthen" your spine by lifting your rib cage and strengthening your abdomen. The improved posture will result in less pressure on painful joints.

Healing Nutrients

With arthritis, eating a healthful variety of foods—including dairy, vegetables and fruits, lentils, soy products, lean meats, and whole grains—can help you boost immunity.

Nearly all nutrients play some role in aiding your body to reduce inflammation and pain. For instance, calcium and magnesium can relax tense muscles. Antioxidants, phytochemicals, lycopenes, and a host of vitamins and minerals are necessary for the synthesis of normal collagen and maintenance of cartilage structures. Some recent National Institutes of Health studies on the efficacy of vitamin B3 show that it improves joint range of motion and reduces pain and swelling. (More on this in Step 5.)

Because some types of inflammatory arthritis are caused when the immune system goes haywire, it makes good sense to do all you can to keep your immune system functioning normally. The mineral zinc—found in meats, seafood (especially oysters), liver, brewer's yeast, milk, beans, and wheat germ—helps strengthen resistance to disease. Other vitamins and minerals needed for the synthesis of normal collagen and maintenance of cartilage structures include vitamins A, B5, B6, zinc, boron, and copper. Patients with rheumatoid arthritis may benefit from supplements of selenium, as it reduces the production of inflammatory prostaglandins and leukotrienes. You can get adequate amounts of these and other important vitamins and minerals by taking a daily vitamin-mineral supplement. Ask your doctor to recommend one that will meet your individual needs.

The Antioxidant Power of Tea.   Both green and black teas are naturally rich sources of flavonoids. These antioxidants neutralize free radicals that can damage the body's cells and lead to disease. Some recent studies indicate that the antioxidants in tea are more potent than those found in many fruits and vegetables. According to a Case Western Reserve University study published in the *Proceedings of the National Academy of Science*, the antioxidants in green tea may prevent and reduce the severity of rheumatoid arthritis. In the study, researchers examined the effects of green tea polyphenols (powerful antioxidants) in collagen-induced arthritis in mice. In each group, scientists found that the mice given green tea polyphenols were less likely to develop arthritis. The arthritic mice that received the green tea polyphenols developed less severe forms of arthritis. While green tea is no substitution for medication, this study may suggest that diet is a key preventive measure in some types of illnesses, including rheumatoid arthritis.

Red Wine May Help Decrease Inflammation.   Some studies identify a compound in red wine that may work to stop arthritis. A scientific paper in the *U.S. Journal of Biological Chemistry* suggests that trans-resveratrol, a natural compound found in red wine, may offer new hope in reducing the pain of arthritis sufferers. A team of researchers found that trans-resveratrol blocks the activation of the gene identified as Cox-2. Considerable evidence has accumulated that Cox-2 is important in creating the inflammation that causes arthritis pain. Trans-resveratrol is a substance produced in the skin of grapes to protect against oxidation and fungal infection caused by external stresses, such as temperature extremes and ultraviolet light. In red wine, trans-resveratrol is found in high concentrations, though its levels vary depending on the particular wine. This natural food substance is the first compound identified that both blocks the Cox-2 gene from being activated and also inactivates the enzyme created by that gene. Some believe that trans-resveratrol may turn out to be an improvement on aspirin in fighting diseases associated with Cox-2, such as arthritis.

Omega-3 Fatty Acids May Reduce Pain. Eating fish such as salmon, mackerel, herring, and sardines, or taking fish oil capsules, may reduce inflammation that stems from arthritis. These fatty acids enable the body to make more products that tend to decrease the inflammation. More than a dozen studies have shown that high doses of fish oil supplements, taken long-term along with pain medication, can reduce joint swelling, ease morning stiffness, and lessen fatigue in people with rheumatoid arthritis. The effective dose may be between three and five grams of the acids daily, although regulated guidelines have not been established regarding supplements of fish oil. Eicosapentaenoic acid (EPA) is available in capsules without a prescription at your drug store or health food store. It is possible to get the recommended amount by making fish an important part of your diet. It takes twelve to sixteen weeks of omega-3 therapy before benefits begin, but check with your doctor before taking a megadose, as it can cause problems for some people.

Vegetarians who want to gain this anti-inflammatory benefit can substitute borage seed oil, flaxseeds or flaxseed oil, or evening primrose oil—all said to be helpful in offsetting the inflammation caused by arthritis.

Lose Weight. Also crucial to reducing pain and staying active with arthritis is maintaining a normal weight, as discussed in Step 5. Studies have shown that obese people, especially older women who are overweight, are at increased risk for knee osteoarthritis. Yet some long-term studies indicate that losing as little as eleven pounds may significantly lower the risk of developing knee osteoarthritis (Framingham Study). Being overweight puts unnecessary weight on aging joints. Some studies show that people who are overweight in their twenties have a greater risk of arthritis later in life.

Mind/Body Exercises

Depending on your perception, your mind can accentuate the pain you feel—or it can diminish it. Using mind/body exercises, you can learn to de-stress the body and turn your focus away from your arthritis pain. A study from the Johns Hopkins School of Medicine concluded that spirituality may be a type of psychological resource that allows people to adjust better to living with a chronic illness. The study, performed on seventy-seven patients with rheumatoid arthritis, concluded that spirituality gave patients a greater sense of meaning and also increased social support—helping them rise to the challenge of a painful, chronic illness. In a similar study done at Duke University, researchers made a similar conclusion, finding that patients who reported being able to control and decrease pain using positive religious and spiritual coping strategies were less likely to experience arthritis joint pain. These patients also had better moods and were more positive in outlook for the future.

Mind/body therapies help distract you from the pain as you focus on something else, such as relaxation, music, breathing, or simply where you are at the moment (mindfulness). I'll explain these therapies and how you can use them each day to decrease stress and pain in Step 6.

Bodywork and Massage

Many women with arthritis find relief with touch therapies such as Swedish massage, the Trager Approach, and the Feldenkrais Method, all discussed in Step 7. Self-massage can be extremely helpful for those with osteoarthritis. For instance, if you have osteoarthritis of the shoulder, massaging your shoulder with soothing salve or liniment may help to ease the pain.

Other touch therapies that may give pain relief include Oriental medical therapies: acupressure, acupuncture, and shiatsu. These ancient healing modalities may help unblock obstructions in the energy flow and allow balance to the body, resulting in reduced pain and healing. For arthritic back pain, chiropractic may offer some relief.

High-Tech Solutions

A host of "gadgets" can help ease arthritis pain by increasing blood flow and circulation to the affected area. They include transcutaneous electrical nerve stimulation (TENS), ultrasound, pulsed galvanic stimulation, electro-acupuncture, and interferential stimulation—all described in Step 8. TENS works by sending electrical impulses to underlying nerve fiber through electrodes placed on the skin.

Older women with severe arthritis of the knees, resulting in a bowlegged stance or walk, may achieve great benefit from custom-molded orthotic devices (lateral wedges) inserted in their shoes. These devices are designed by a physician in collaboration with an orthotic specialist and are made specifically for individual patients to "open" the medial joint space/compartments and bring the stance toward a more normal appearance.

In some cases, if nonsurgical treatments fail, surgery may be necessary to remove bone or joint tissue, to fuse joints, or do a total joint replacement. Surgery can replace damaged cartilage in order to ease arthritis pain. Some of these procedures are briefly explained in Step 8, but your doctor can advise you if this the next step for you. Additionally, surgery may be needed in some cases of severe refractory carpal tunnel syndrome. However, refractory milder cases may respond to laser acupuncture.

When to Call the Doctor

If you have arthritis pain that is moderate to severe—persistent or progressive—you should call your doctor. This should be done immediately if you are unable to do your normal activities because of the arthritis, or if you have associated significant joint swelling, tenderness, redness, heat, fever, significant weight loss, or changes in strength or sensation.

CHAPTER EIGHT

Osteoporosis

"It happened suddenly when I bent down to pick up the newspaper," Judith said. "I felt this excruciating pain in my back that kept me from standing upright. Then with every step I took, the pain worsened. I called my husband, who took me to a nearby emergency room. After taking an X ray, the ER doctor said I had a spinal fracture, and she ordered a bone density test. That's how I found out I had osteoporosis."

Lisa's story was pretty much the same: "I suffered my first fracture when I tripped over my son's bicycle on the driveway. At first I thought my foot was sprained and wrapped it in an athletic bandage. However, by the next day, I could not put any weight on it, so my friend drove me to a nearby outpatient clinic. After an X ray and bone density test, the clinic doctor told me I had the bone density of a woman twenty years older."

Judith's and Lisa's stories would not sound unusual except that both women were in their mid-forties when they were diagnosed with osteoporosis, a painful and debilitating disease that strikes millions each year. Osteoporosis, meaning "porous bones," causes bones to become so brittle and weak that simply bending over to pick up a child, carrying a heavy purse or briefcase, or even coughing can result in a painful fracture.

Just two decades ago, osteoporosis was thought to be a normal result of aging, like wrinkles or gray hair, a disease of older women, particularly those over sixty. Nevertheless, newer information shows that this disease should be a concern of all women, no matter what their age.

The statistics are frightening. Osteoporosis affects more than 30 million Americans—mostly women, although men can get it, too. This painful disease affects half of all women over the age of forty-five, and 90 percent of women over age seventy-five. It is the most common cause of all fractures, and the twelfth leading cause of death in the United States.

With aging America, millions of women are now hitting fifty, making this the largest group of women to go through menopause in our nation's history and almost guaranteeing that the number of fractures will increase as well. The good news is that you can reduce or even prevent painful fractures altogether, using the latest therapies available.

What Is Osteoporosis?

Osteoporosis is thinning of the bones, or a decrease in the density of the bone. As your bones become thinner, they become easier to fracture or break. For millions of older adults, mostly women, such daily activities as standing, walking, and bending may be enough to cause a broken bone. These fractures commonly occur in the back, the hip, the foot, and the wrist. In fact, I've seen patients whose seemingly minor incidents, such as stumbling over a rug, result in a fracture with severe pain, limitation, and expense.

What You Might Feel: Signs and Symptoms

Building strong bones during childhood and adolescence is the best defense against developing painful fractures later on in life. In fact, by about age twenty, the average woman has acquired 98 percent of her skeletal mass.

Ages and Stages. Osteoporosis begins to start its damage at about age thirty to forty. During this time the removal of bone begins to equal the building of bone. After age forty, the total amount of bone becomes less. At this time, the removal of bone continues at a much faster pace than bone-building, and osteoporosis is detectable on a bone density test. Still, even though you may know osteoporosis is present, there are usually no signs or symptoms that you can feel.

Between ages forty-five and fifty-five, bone loss occurs at varying degrees. For instance, I have patients who are in their fifties with extremely strong bones and no signs of osteoporosis, and some patients as young as thirty-five with early signs of the disease who must take medication to try to boost bone density. One thirty-five-year-old mother of two small children was recently diagnosed with osteoporosis after suffering a cracked rib during a coughing spell. You may lose bone faster or slower than others, depending on your risk factors.

Thin Bones Lead to Painful Fractures.   As osteoporosis continues its destruction, your bones will eventually become thin enough that they break or fracture. You might trip over a crack in the sidewalk and suffer a fractured ankle. Or lifting a bag of potting soil may result in a wrist fracture. One woman I saw recently suffered a spinal fracture after leaning over to pick up her three-year-old grandson.

As the fractures continue, your pain will escalate, even setting you up for disability. Deformities in your spine (called a dowager's hump) and other areas may become much more obvious. You may have more difficulty getting around and doing daily activities because of the pain and stiffness. The good news is that this stage is becoming less common, as treatment for osteoporosis has become available to prevent future fractures.

What Causes Osteoporosis?

Our bones are complex, living tissue. Up until a certain age, the body constantly breaks down old bone and rebuilds new bone, a process called "remodeling." During childhood and adolescence, more bone is built than removed, so bones become larger and stronger. At a certain point, the amount of bone removed catches up with the amount of bone built, and osteoporosis disrupts the natural bone-building cycle, resulting in a decrease in the total amount of bone.

At menopause, a decline in estrogen speeds up the removal of bone. During the five to ten years after menopause, there is accelerated bone loss. In fact, women have a *40 percent chance* of having a fracture at some time by age fifty, and many women have lost a startling 25 percent of their bone density within the first five years after menopause. This may be difficult to comprehend for active women in midlife, when we often take good health for granted. However, at this life stage, it is estimated that less than 10 percent of those who have osteoporosis actually know they have it, and do not learn of it until they fracture a bone!

If the decline in bone continues over a period of ten to twenty years, bones become thinner, weaker, and easier to break or fracture. When this happens, there will be pain from the fracture. While usually the first break will eventually heal, as long as the bones are thin and weak they will be increasingly susceptible to more fractures, resulting in immobility or even death.

If fractures only happened to fingers or toes, this would be inconvenient but not very limiting. But osteoporosis does not commonly affect fingers and toes. Instead, it attacks with painful and disfiguring fractures on those specific bones that allow us to be active and enjoy life: the bones of the spine, the wrist, the shoulder, and the hip. These fractures cause severe limitation and can also cause deformities, especially when they affect the spine.

While experts used to recommend guarding against osteoporosis *after* menopause, new research shows that bone loss can and must be treated *long before fractures and deformity occur.* In other words, no woman should have to suffer from a bone fracture, dowager's hump, or loss of height . . . if you take prevention measures early in life.

KNOW YOUR RISK

Risk Factors That Cannot Be Changed

- Genetic predisposition: Osteoporosis appears to run in families. If your mother or grandmother had osteoporosis, your chances of getting it are increased.
- Race: Caucasians and Asian women are at greater risk of getting osteoporosis, although Hispanic and African American women have a significant risk.
- Sex and age: Women have a higher risk than men, and bone weakness increases with age.
- History of fractures after age forty: If you have had a fracture in early or middle adulthood, this may show susceptibility to fractures or less dense bones and increase your chance of getting osteoporosis.

Risk Factors That Can Be Changed

- Lack of regular exercise: Exercise, particularly weight-bearing exercise, is necessary to stimulate and strengthen bone.

- Smoking: Women who smoke have lower levels of estrogen compared to nonsmokers and frequently go through menopause earlier.
- Being underweight: Small-boned women are at greatest risk for osteoporosis.
- Heavy alcohol consumption: Alcohol's detrimental effect on bone tissue possibly results in reduced bone formation. Mineral and hormonal metabolism can also be impaired with alcohol consumption.
- Medications: Certain medications, such as glucocorticoids, thyroid medication, anticonvulsants, and antacids containing aluminum, increase your risk. Medications used to treat endometriosis (gonadotropin-releasing hormones or GnRH) also increase the risk of osteoporosis.
- Low calcium in diet: Because bones need calcium to stay strong, low dietary calcium results in less dense bones.
- Menopause: Bone losses increases dramatically with the reduction of the hormone estrogen at menopause. Using a combination of lifestyle changes and medications, if necessary, you can stop this loss from happening altogether.
- Being athletic: Women who vigorously exercise, such as long distance runners and gymnasts, make skip menstrual periods. The reduced estrogen production can result in osteoporosis.

RED FLAG!

If you have osteoporosis, problems that make falls more likely can increase the risk of hip fractures. Weakness when walking, unsteadiness, dizziness, medications that cause lightheadedness, alcohol use, and heart problems may all contribute to further falls and hip fracture. Tripping over objects in the home or workplace greatly raises the risk of hip fracture. Telephone cords, slippery rugs, rooms darkened by low lighting, especially at night, can add to the chances of falling.

HOW IS OSTEOPOROSIS DIAGNOSED?

It's important to know that it is *never too late* to try to prevent fractures, but the most important fracture to prevent is the first one. To find out if you are at risk for osteoporosis, have your bone mineral density (BMD) evaluated, as this is the best method for determining whether a person has osteoporosis or is at risk of developing it. BMD testing is a quick, noninvasive, and accurate method for assessing future fracture risk. Bone density tests (often referred to as a DEXA test), which are fast, painless, and safe, measure the bone density in your spine, hip, and/or wrist, the most common sites of fractures due to osteoporosis. Some newer bone density tests measure bone density in your heel or shinbone and in your middle finger.

All bone density measurements are compared to two norms: (1) the expected bone density of someone your age, sex, and size; and (2) the optimal peak bone density of a healthy young adult of the same sex. Once your doctor obtains these scores, treatment will be given, if necessary. If detected at this early point, specific steps, including the use of bone-building medications, can be taken to slow or stop the disease, and thus prevent the first fracture. However, if osteoporosis continues undetected, the bones gradually grow thinner over the years until a serious injury occurs. Because everyone's experience with this disease is different, bone loss occurs at varying rates. This makes it even more important to find out your own bone density to see if you are at a higher risk. If your bone density is in a good range, then you can use the easy steps for prevention outlined in my 8-step program. If treatment is needed, you can get started with this, as well. Talk to your doctor about a bone density test and to see if treatment is necessary.

Treating Osteoporosis Pain

Taking measures to build strong bones, especially before the age of thirty, is the best defense against osteoporosis, and a healthy lifestyle, including a diet high in bone-boosting calcium and vitamin D, along with daily weight-bearing exercise, is critically important for keeping bones strong. Resistance and high-impact exercise adds to the improvement of high peak bone mass and may even help to prevent falls in older women.

Medications

Most of the medications used for back and arthritis pain are helpful for treating the pain of fractures. These include analgesics, non-steroid anti-inflammatory drugs (NSAIDs), and narcotic and non-narcotic pain medications, among others. But along with healing the fracture, it's important to make this fracture *your last*, and you do that by building bone density and strengthening the bones you have.

If you are menopausal, this is the time when bone loss occurs with the reduction in the hormone estrogen. While your doctor may recommend hormone replacement therapy (HRT), treatment that aims to partially restore the hormones that naturally decrease as you enter menopause, a groundbreaking study published in the July 2002 issue of the *Journal of the American Medical Association* confirms that the risks of taking HRT far outweigh the benefits. The HRT study was one part of the Women's Health Initiative (WHI), which was started in 1991 by the National Institutes of Health. With 160,000 women participating, WHI is considered the largest study of women's health ever. Researchers halted the HRT study early after noting an increase in the incidence of breast cancer and heart disease.

Talk to your doctor about your health history to see if hormone replacement therapy is for you. If not, there are other effective medications, including the bone-building biphosphonates such as Fosamax (alendronate), Actonel (residronate), or Didronel (etidronate) that significantly increase bone density. As bone density improves, the risk of painful fractures decreases. Calcitonin is another medication that is available to slow bone removal, which should help to improve the bone density. This medication, which is available as a nasal spray, is often recommended for women more than five years after menopause who do not choose to take hormone replacement therapy. Evista (raloxifene) is one of a new group of medications called SERMS, that are used to build bone in osteoporosis. The advantage of raloxifene is that it doesn't increase the risk of breast cancer, which is why many women choose not to take estrogen at menopause. Raloxifene also does not cause uterine bleeding and irregular menstrual periods, which often occur with hormone replacement therapy.

NEW TREATMENT

There's hope for new treatment for osteoporosis in near future. Scientists believe that within five years, a treatment given once a year may be enough to prevent osteoporosis and painful fractures. The study, in the February 28, 2002 issue of the *New England Journal of Medicine*, was on a drug called Zometa (zoledronic acid), a bisphosphonate that is given to cancer patients to treat problems in which calcium leaches from the bones. If subsequent studies are conclusive, men and women may be able to get an annual osteoporosis shot—just like they get their yearly flu vaccine.

Natural Cures

It is estimated that one-third of all persons sixty years old and older suffer falls each year—falls that lead to painful, debilitating fractures. It makes sense that if you have experienced one fracture and have thinning bones, it takes less impact for a subsequent fall to cause another fracture. That's why it's important to prevent falls altogether using these natural self-care tips:

- Have your vision checked annually.
- Wear sturdy shoes with nonskid soles.
- Limit alcohol consumption.
- Make sure you know the side effects of any medications taken.
- If you smoke, quit.
- Improve safety measures at home and work, avoiding places where you might trip or fall.
- Make sure you have adequate lighting to avoid tripping or slipping.
- Have grab bars installed by your toilet and tub.
- Use nonskid mats in the tub or shower.
- Firmly attach carpets and rugs.
- Use stair railings to help you stay balanced.

Exercise

Focus on Weight-bearing Exercise.　　Weight-bearing exercises, specifically walking, aerobics, racket sports, and strenuous strength training, are crucial to increasing bone mass. This type of activity puts vertical force on the bones. This force creates mini-electrical currents that help strengthen the bone being stressed. Some of the best bone-building exercises, described in detail in Step 4, include the following: aerobics (low-impact), biking, dancing, rowing, running, skating, stair-climbing, strength training, and walking.

Tai Chi.　　Can you stand on one foot without losing your balance? If you've had a fracture, consider doing Tai Chi. It may reduce your fear of falling as you become stronger and more physically balanced.

Tai Chi, an ancient Chinese martial art in which you follow a series of slow, graceful movements that mimic the movements in daily living, is highly recommended for women with osteoporosis. Studies have found that engaging in this discipline may reduce the risk of falling, and therefore the risk of fracture. Researchers have suggested that Tai Chi helps improve your balance as the exercises focus on slow, continuous movement.

Healing Nutrients

To keep bones strong, be sure to get enough calcium and vitamin D in your daily diet, as discussed in Step 5. There are many foods high in calcium, including vegetables and soy products, which are low in fat. Researchers believe that soy might be considered a "wonder food" when it comes to building bone strength. In the body, the isoflavones found in soy foods are converted into phytoestrogens, or plant compounds that mimic estrogen, although they are a lot weaker than human estrogen (about 500 to 1,000 times weaker). While the isoflavones look and act like estrogen in the body, unlike estrogen they are not linked with cancer.

In osteoporosis research, the isoflavones genistein and daidzein, two components of the soybean, have been shown to inhibit bone breakdown in animals because of their estrogenlike actions. Research published in *Obstetrics and Gynecology* suggests that a soy-rich diet may reduce the risk of painful fractures. In the Japanese study, researchers found that women in early and late post-menopausal stages who consumed the most soy foods, including tofu, soymilk, and soybeans, had significantly denser bones than women who consumed the least soy foods. The women who ate the soy-rich diet also had fewer backaches and aching joints.

Mind/Body Exercises

If you have been diagnosed with osteoporosis and are experiencing pain and immobility, mind/body exercises can help you keep the illness in perspective during the healing process. Be sure to review the discussions on the relaxation response, music therapy, deep abdominal breathing, and visualization in chapter 14, as these exercises can help you to replace negative thoughts with a more optimistic, hopeful mind-set.

Bodywork and Massage

The following bodywork techniques, explained in Step 7, appear to have healing results for those with osteoporosis, especially as you learn to de-stress and become more aware of your posture and positioning.

- Trager: gentle and nonintrusive movements that produce deep relaxation, increase flexibility and mobility, and relieve pain
- Feldenkrais Method: movement therapy and gentle hands-on massage that helps arthritis patients expand their range of motion and improve their breathing
- Rolfing/Structural Integration: a system of body restructuring and movement that focuses on the myofascia, the connective tissue that surrounds muscles, to release tension

Chiropractic is another hands-on therapy that may give some pain relief. This discipline relies on manipulation of the spine and muscles, in conjunction with nutrition and exercise. Spinal manipulation or adjustment attempts to relieve pain by increasing the mobility between spinal vertebrae that have become restricted or locked or out of position. These manipulations can be gentle stretching or pressure, repeated minor motions, or a few high-velocity thrusts.

High-Tech Solutions

Using a TENS (Transcutaneous Electrical Nerve Stimulation) unit may help alleviate some of the discomfort you might have from fractures. If you have back pain from a compression fracture of a vertebral body in your spine, then you may be a candidate for percutaneous vertebroplasty, which involves infusing a cementlike substance into the fractured area. Your doctor can guide you on this procedure.

When to Call the Doctor

Anytime you have pain and do not know the cause, call your doctor for an evaluation. Osteoporosis causes painful fractures, but the disease is also silent, especially as it quietly destroys your bones. The next time you see your doctor, ask about a bone density test, described in Step 1, to see if it is necessary at your age and life stage. Then follow the recommendations in this chapter to keep your bones strong—no matter what your age.

PART III

Dr. Smith's Holistic Program to End Pain

CHAPTER NINE

Step 1: Start with an Accurate Diagnosis

Pain has always been an elusive phenomenon. Especially with women, pain encompasses your entire being—your physical sensation and emotional perception—and affects all aspects of your life. Despite scientists' trying to separate mind and body, it cannot be done with chronic pain. For instance, at our clinic, after I do the initial physical examination and discussion, my patients are often thoroughly evaluated by other specialists—including a psychologist, neurologist, physical medicine rehabilitation specialist, and a physical therapist—so we can get the most complete picture of the cause of pain and how it can best be treated. When evaluations are completed, I meet or talk with this team of health care professionals about each patient's case. Because we gather facts about the complex nature of the patient's pain—and each patient is different—I can then prescribe a complete multifaceted, individualized treatment program that includes effective medications, specific exercises, dietary changes, stress management, and a focus on changing lifestyle habits.

Choosing a Pain Specialist

Your doctor plays the first major role in determining the precise source of your pain, as well as testing to see if the problem is isolated or is associated with a serious illness. Not only does he or she serve as the one who can accurately diagnose and prescribe treatment for the pain, this health care professional may become a close, dependable friend to talk to when concerns turn into ongoing worries and anxieties.

Trust Is an Important Factor

Because of managed care, finding the right person to diagnose and treat pain-related problems properly and cost-effectively is not always easy. That's why you must carefully choose a physician whom you can trust to know your medical history and take responsibility for your overall health care. Then, as a rule, if your response to initial treatment for pain is unsatisfactory and the lack of good control of symptoms still interferes with your quality of life, you need to see a specialist. (If you are in a health maintenance organization (HMO), you may need to ask your gatekeeper or primary care physician for a referral to a specialist. Carefully read your policy manual to find out.)

Find a Board Certified Specialist

Make sure the health care professional you choose is board certified in his or her specialty and has experience and/or special training in pain management. To be board certified, the doctor has completed four years of premedical education in a college or university, four years of medical school resulting in an medical doctor or doctor of osteopathy degree, and at least three years of specialty training in an accredited residency program.

Here are some of the doctors who specialize in pain management for women:

• *Pain specialists*, who are given credentials by the American Board of Anesthesiology collaboratively with the American Board of Physical Medicine and Rehabilitation and the American Board of Psychiatry and Neurology, or the American Academy of Pain Medicine, and are usually board certified anesthesiologists, neurologists, physiatrists, psychiatrists, or oncologists with additional training in pain management.

• *Neurologists*, who diagnose and treat disorders of the nervous system, including common pain problems such as headaches, back pain, muscle disorders, and neuropathy (carpal tunnel syndrome), among others.

● *Gynecologists*, who diagnose and treat disorders of the women's reproductive system, including common pain problems such as premenstrual syndrome (PMS), menstrual cramps, pelvic pain, breast pain, endometriosis, and ovarian cysts, among others.

● *Rheumatologists*, who diagnose and treat arthritis and other diseases of the joints, muscles, and bones, including rheumatoid arthritis, osteoarthritis, gout, lupus, back pain, osteoporosis, fibromyalgia, bursitis, and tendonitis.

● *Orthopedists*, who specialize in the diagnosis, clinical treatment, and surgical repair of bone injuries and treat muscle problems and joint tissues (tendons, ligaments, cartilage).

● *Otolaryngologists*, who diagnose and treat disorders of the ears, nose, and throat, including common pain problems such as sinusitis, earache, headache, TMJ, and chronic sore throat, among others.

● *Podiatrists*, who specialize in diagnosis and clinical and surgical care for foot and leg problems, including correcting improper alignments of the feet and legs with orthotics (shoe inserts).

● *Psychologists* who diagnose and do therapy for problems associated with pain, perception, and emotional issues.

Questions You May Ask

In choosing a pain specialist, some women ask friends for recommendations, check the physician's credentials, or call the local hospital for referrals. In this age of managed care, you will need to check the list of doctors who will accept your insurance provider. Nevertheless, none of these methods is "foolproof" for finding a qualified professional with whom you can feel comfortable.

One of the most important factors when choosing this health care professional is paying attention to your personal likes and dislikes. Do you feel more comfortable with a man or woman? Should your physician be older than you, the same age, or younger? Do you have a preference as to educational background? These questions are important to consider when making your selection.

Ask the following questions as you go through the process of choosing a pain specialist:

- Is the doctor board certified?
- Where did the doctor go to medical school? (Your local medical society can provide this information too.)
- Is the doctor involved in any academic pursuits, such as teaching, writing, or research? This doctor may be more up-to-date in the latest developments in his field.
- Where does the doctor have hospital privileges and where are these hospitals located? Some doctors may not admit patients to certain hospitals, and this is an important consideration for those with chronic health problems.
- Does the doctor accept your particular type of health insurance, or is the doctor a member of the medical panel associated with your HMO?

Make sure the doctor's office hours fit with your daily schedule. How is payment made? What insurance providers are accepted? Ask for information about emergency availability and charges. Is your doctor always on call or are other doctors sharing in this? Even the receptionist's responses might set the tone and help you decide if this is the right office. The support staff will be the ones who help you most with prescriptions, obtaining necessary lab work and X rays, and making appointments with hospitals or other professional services.

Changes in medical coverage may mean that the doctor you now see will not be the one you see in a year or two. This makes it even more important to understand your particular problem fully, stay abreast of treatment methods, and fully follow the management plan as discussed in this book.

Plan a Consultation

Plan an initial consultation with the doctor during which you can get to know each other. This will include a detailed interview and physical examination. Ease of patient-physician communication is important to receive the highest quality of care and comfort needed during anxious moments.

If you've identified the type of pain you have in chapters 3 through 8, read over the specific tests in this chapter. I will explain which test is used to diagnose a problem, what you will feel, the precautions, the pros and cons, and how you can help your doctor by interpreting the message of pain symptoms to get the best diagnosis and most effective treatment.

Write Down All Concerns

Before I order the appropriate tests, I need to know all about my patient and her symptoms. I ask my patients to bring a list of concerns with them to each consultation. Many times women are hesitant to say exactly how they feel or how the pain has impacted their lives. One patient, Linda, age thirty-seven, whose husband had convinced her that her chronic pelvic pain was an excuse to get out of family responsibilities. This mother of four lived with debilitating pain for two years before finally seeking answers. At the consultation, Linda described a triad of symptoms, including painful menstruation (dysmenorrhea), painful intercourse (dyspareunia), and painful bowel movements (dyskysia). She also had severe pelvic pain during ovulation and menstruation. Two previous doctors had misdiagnosed her with irritable bowel syndrome because diarrhea and constipation, along with intestinal pain, are related to menstruation. I assured Linda that her pain was very real, and after doing a physical exam and running some diagnostic tests, I found a cyst with the "ground glass" appearance of an endometrioma. At that point, I suspected endometriosis, an overgrowth of the endometrium outside the uterus, which causes chronic pain. After laparoscopy to diagnose the problem and remove the scar tissue, along with a combination of medications, Linda's pain diminished, and she was able to reclaim her active life. She exuded greater confidence in follow-up visits because someone finally believed that she was not overreacting to the pain she felt.

To get an accurate diagnosis, be sure to write down and bring to your visit the following personal facts:

- Any health concerns
- Symptoms you've noticed
- Past illnesses and medications
- Medications you are taking now; medications you've taken in the past
- Questions you have about your health and pain
- Your family history of illnesses
- Lifestyle habits (diet, exercise, smoking)
- Main causes of stress in your life

Also, bring with you all medications, vitamins, and supplements that you are taking. Your doctor can let you know which ones are safe—and which may not be used safely.

Give Your Medical History

The specialist you choose will seek an accurate diagnosis by obtaining a detailed personal medical history, including information on symptoms, your activity level and diet, your home and work environment, and family medical history, and then doing a thorough medical examination.

During this evaluation, it is important that you talk openly with your doctor to interpret the overall results of the total discussion, including the physical examination, the laboratory testing, and X rays or other diagnostic tests. This will allow you to have a firm understanding of your pain problem and will be the basis for the treatment plan. Some questions your doctor may ask include:

- Where does it hurt?
- Can you describe the pain? (Pinching, throbbing, pressure, burning, crushing, piercing)
- When did the problem start?
- Is it the result of an injury?
- What other symptoms do you have?
- Does the pain stay the same or does it come and go?
- Have you had the problem before?
- How badly does it hurt on a scale of 0 to 10? (0 being not at all; 10 being unbearable)
- Have you had a previous diagnosis?
- Have you had medical treatment for the problem?
- Have you undergone unusual stress?
- Have you had surgery?
- Were you in an accident?

During the physical examination, your doctor will particularly focus on the area of your pain. Your doctor will look for the following:

- Obvious swelling
- Inflamed tissue or joint
- Redness or discoloration
- Loss of function
- Abnormal appearance

- Tenderness
- Loss of range of motion
- Unusual lump, knot, or bulge

Solving the Mystery of Pain

No matter what type pain you have, your doctor will act like a medical "detective," trying to solve the pain mystery. For example, in the case of headache pain, your doctor will first perform a detailed examination of your head and neck, the muscular strength and movement, sensation, balance testing, and reflex testing. The doctor will also need information and facts, such as when you experience this pain, what symptoms coincide with it (such as blurred vision, nausea, or irritability), how this correlates with your menstrual cycle, medications you are taking, and any stressors you are experiencing, among others. The best way to help your doctor to solve the problem and to make an accurate diagnosis is to totally understand your pain—how it feels, when it happens, and what helps to resolve it.

Your doctor will also ask how the pain interferes with your everyday life including:

- Household activities
- Work/career
- Concentrating
- Doing hobbies/leisure activities
- Social activities
- Walking
- Relationships with spouse/family/friends
- Sex

Depending on the physical examination and discussion, your doctor will then decide which tests are appropriate to give an accurate diagnosis and to ensure that no other medical problems are present. Because each patient is different, your testing may be significantly different from anyone else's, depending on your pain symptoms and findings made during the physical examination and discussion. In other words, just because your best friend had an ultrasound for her pelvic pain does not mean that you will also need that same test.

If you fear one specific diagnosis, such as bone cancer, be sure you tell your doctor. After the diagnosis, if you still do not feel comfortable with the outcome, talk to your doctor and then have more testing. Or, get a second opinion until you have peace of mind that the problem has been diagnosed correctly. Then, proper treatment can begin.

Once the problem is properly identified, your doctor will prescribe a treatment regimen that can help relieve the pain. If the laboratory and imaging tests are negative, do not give up hope. That doesn't mean your pain doesn't exist. For instance, there is no available test to diagnose fibromyalgia. Whether the cause of your pain can be identified or not, continue to seek treatment and stay on the 8-step program until you experience relief from the pain and the resulting emotional issues.

Common Laboratory Tests

Depending on your symptoms and discussion, your doctor will start by ordering laboratory tests, as well as other diagnostic scans or X rays. Sometimes the tests are ordered so your doctor can exclude more serious medical problems. In most cases, the tests can generally all be done in one visit to the laboratory.

Complete Blood Count

A complete blood count (CBC) is a standard laboratory test for all pain disorders and is used to find common blood disorders and to evaluate your overall health. A CBC measures the hemoglobin, red cells, white cells, and platelets and can also find many of the common blood disorders, such as anemia, which can cause fatigue and tiredness.

The chemistries in your blood will also be checked along with the CBC and will usually include kidney and liver tests, cholesterol and other fats in the blood, and calcium levels.

Routine Screening Tests for Women

Depending on your age, symptoms, and health history, other routine screening tests may include any and all of the following:

- Blood pressure monitoring
- Urine testing
- Pelvic exam with Pap smear
- Colon cancer screening and rectal exam

- Chest X ray
- Mammogram
- Bone density test (to screen for osteoporosis)
- For those over 35, a baseline electrocardiogram

Other Diagnostic Lab Tests

Serum Hormone Analysis

The serum hormone analysis is used to assess imbalances, which can lead to problems such as menstrual irregularities, premenstrual syndrome (PMS), pelvic pain, and headaches. A key to proper functioning of the menstrual cycle is balanced estrogen and progesterone. The cyclic rhythm is created by the regular highs and lows of these hormones each month. When one or both hormones are imbalanced, you may experience a host of problems, including menstrual irregularity and subsequent pain, headache, and PMS.

During the forties, these hormones naturally decline. Usually progesterone is the first hormone to be deficient. When estrogen declines, the menstrual periods stop. A serum hormone blood test can assess your total estrogen, total progesterone, sex-hormone-binding globulin (SHBG), total testosterone, total cholesterol, and HDL ("good") and LDL ("bad") cholesterol.

Thyroid Stimulating Hormone (TSH) Test

The thyroid stimulating hormone test is a standard blood test for most adult women and is used to help determine treatment for some hormonal problems and menstrual disorders. Thyroid disease is very common, especially in women and those with a strong family history of the disease. The problem for those who suffer with menstrual disorders and subsequent pain is that thyroid disease can interfere with ovarian function. The TSH test is easy, relatively cheap, and can lead to an accurate diagnosis of thyroid disease so that therapy can be started early on when it has the best chance of working.

The TSH level does not vary with the stage of your menstrual cycle or time of day, so the test is performed at any time. Unless the TSH level returns as abnormal, there is no reason for further thyroid testing. If the TSH is abnormal, then the test should be repeated with a measurement of free thyroxine (Free T4). In most patients, a high TSH (more than 4 to 5 IU/L, depending on the lab) signals an underactive thyroid (hypothyroidism). Suppressed levels of TSH usually indicate an overactive thyroid (hyperthyroidism).

Erythrocyte Sedimentation Rate, Rheumatoid Factor, and Anti-Nuclear Antibody Tests

Erythrocyte sedimentation rate (sed rate), rheumatoid factor, and anti-nuclear antibody (ANA) are blood tests your doctor may order if arthritis or inflammatory disease is suspected.

Erythrocyte sedimentation rate (sed rate or ESR) is a test that gives a rough index of inflammation. In rheumatoid arthritis, systemic lupus erythematosus (SLE or lupus), and other similar types of inflammatory arthritis, this test may be abnormal. Yet in osteoarthritis and fibromyalgia, the sed rate is usually normal. The sed rate is not specific and can be elevated if you have some infection, a tumor, diabetes, liver disease, or are pregnant.

Rheumatoid factor is a blood test that measures an abnormal protein in the blood and is positive in 70 to 80 percent of patients with rheumatoid arthritis. However, this blood test may be positive in healthy people and negative in people with rheumatoid arthritis, so it is not conclusive.

Anti-nuclear antibody (ANA) is a blood test that checks for an abnormal protein in the blood that is commonly found with systemic lupus erythematosus. Lupus is a type of arthritis that is common in younger women and can cause great pain and fatigue, as well as kidney disease, heart disease, or brain disorders. More than 90 percent of lupus patients have a positive blood test for anti-nuclear antibody. Again, ANA can be positive in those who do not have lupus or in those with unrelated diseases. The ANA test is important, but your doctor will want to look for other clues you might have before making a diagnosis.

Joint Fluid Test

A joint fluid test is done to determine if the cause of pain is arthritis, including osteoarthritis, rheumatoid arthritis, gout, and infectious arthritis, among others. Different types of arthritis may cause changes in the joint fluid. Most arthritis causes swelling in the joints, which is a result of excess fluid production or swelling of the joint lining. Removing a sample of the joint fluid with a small needle under local anesthesia can be a quick, safe, and almost painless and inexpensive way to quickly find out what's causing joint pain.

Normal joints contain a very small amount of joint fluid, and it's usually a yellow, almost clear, and somewhat thick (viscous) fluid that drips slowly from a needle.

With osteoarthritis, the joint fluid usually looks normal (not viscous or cloudy), but there is an increased amount. With rheumatoid arthritis (inflammatory arthritis), the fluid is usually more cloudy and thinner, and there is also more fluid than normal. With gout, the fluid is often cloudy and has crystals in it, which can be seen under a special polarized microscope. In infectious arthritis in the joints, a sample of joint fluid will allow your doctor to diagnose the infection that could damage or even destroy the joint if left untreated.

Imaging Tests

Using the results of your medical history, physical examination, and routine or specific blood tests, your doctor may order one of the following high-tech diagnostic tools to confirm a diagnosis or to eliminate more serious problems.

X rays

X rays are one radiographic tool used to assess joint pain, back pain, sports injuries, broken bones, bone spurs, fractures, cancer, and some infections, as well as to rule out other serious problems. Your doctor may use X rays for osteoarthritis, inflammatory types of arthritis, bursitis, tendonitis, fibromyalgia, carpal tunnel, sprains and strains, among others. (Note: X rays cannot detect a ruptured disc.)

Since X rays were discovered in 1895 by German physicist Wilhelm Konrad Roentgen, they have been one of the most important diagnostic tools in medicine. Even though the new ultrasound (high-frequency sound) and other radiographic techniques have since been developed, a majority of medical imaging is still done with X rays.

An X ray exposes your body to a small amount of radiation to produce an image of the internal organs. As the X ray enters the body, it is absorbed differently depending on the organ or bone. For example, your ribs absorb much radiation and appear white on the image. Your lungs do not absorb as much radiation and appear darker.

The procedure: You will be given a gown to wear and instructed to remove any jewelry or glasses. The technician will have you either lie down or stand up and position you against the film (which looks like a large board) so that accurate pictures can be taken (usually a front and side view). You will be completely still while the technician leaves the room and turns on the machine to take the image. When the radiographic equipment is activated, a beam of X ray goes through your body to expose the film. The technician may have you move into various positions to get different views, and then will take the film to a lab to be developed. The film is read by a radiologist, a doctor who is trained to read radiographic film. After the radiologist analyzes the X rays, your doctor will be sent a written evaluation, and your doctor will give you the results.

What you might feel: During the X ray, you may have to move your body in various positions and hold them until the X ray is taken. If an X ray is being taken of the cervical spine (neck), you may have to hold your mouth open wide so the technician can capture the upper part of the spine behind the teeth. Some awkward positions may be uncomfortable, but it is only for a short period of time. Because X rays are invisible, the electromagnetic radiation creates no sensation when it passes through the body.

The precautions: Be sure to let your doctor know if there is any chance you might be pregnant.

The upside: For some types of acute pain, X rays can give a fast evaluation of the problem so your doctor can prescribe treatment immediately. Because an X ray is an inexpensive method of assessing internal problems, it is easily accessible at most doctor's offices and outpatient centers.

The downside: It's important to limit the number of X rays you have taken in order to avoid overexposure to radiation, which may lead to cancer. Also, X rays are not effective for diagnosing soft tissue pain or small tumors in the bones.

The bottom line: X ray imaging is the fastest and easiest way for a physician to view and assess broken bones, cracked skull, and injured backbone. Because imaging is fast and efficient, it is useful for emergency situations. You will usually have the results back within a day.

Magnetic Resonance Imaging (MRI)

Magnetic imaging is used to diagnose back pain, headache, TMJ, tendonitis, carpal tunnel syndrome, torn ligaments, damaged cartilage, fractures, ruptured disc or disc disease, infections, and tumors, among many other things. Unlike X rays, which emit radioactive beams, MRI can be safely used to assess problems with the female reproductive system, pelvis, hips, and bladder. However, expectant mothers are advised to avoid MRIs during the first twelve weeks of pregnancy.

Magnetic resonance imaging (MRI) uses radio waves and a powerful magnet to gather accurate information about internal organs and tissues. Then a computer uses this information to generate realistic pictures that represent your body. MRI can evaluate musculoskeletal, soft tissue, and joint problems and find abnormalities of cartilage and ligaments that routine X rays cannot. This imaging test can often reveal the cause of severe back pain, and can show osteoarthritis and other types of arthritis, as well as ruptured discs. MRI may also be used to diagnose cancer, as well as heart and vascular diseases.

The procedure: With the older type of MRI, you lie on your back on a flat table that is moved back and forth inside the MRI tunnel, a long nonmagnetic tube. You will have to hold your breath for a few seconds at a time while the technician takes the picture. This entire procedure takes from 30 to 60 minutes to complete.

What you might feel: The older, conventional type of MRI is a closed cylinder-shaped magnet, and it may cause you to feel claustrophobic. Ask your doctor about the new "open" MRIs that are open partially or on all sides. Some new MRIs are wider and do not fully enclose the patient. While the newer models allow for more patient comfort, the images may not be as precise as with conventional MRIs, so work with your doctor to find the best outcome.

With some MRIs, your doctor will hook up an intravenous line ahead of time for a contrast dye to be administered about halfway through the imaging test so areas of abnormality or inflammation are easier to detect. While this dye is different from contrast dyes used for X ray, and reactions are not common, if you have *any* allergies, make sure your doctor knows this ahead of time before the MRI is scheduled. You will have to sign a release prior to this procedure as a precautionary measure to protect medical personnel from liability should you have any type of reaction.

Precautions: Because of the MRI's tremendous magnetic field, if you have a metal object implanted in your body, such as an IUD, metal pins, surgical screws, or even braces, the MRI may pull on that object, resulting in a distorted image. Even a tattoo or permanent eyeliner can potentially cause a problem, and tooth fillings may distort the image of the facial area or the brain. Let your doctor know *before* the MRI is scheduled if you have such an object implanted inside your body, and take off all jewelry prior to the test. Also, if your doctor uses the conventional, closed-in MRI, ask about an anti-anxiety medication, which can help alleviate excessive fears.

The upside: An MRI does not have the radiation exposure of CT scan or X ray. While it can show some problems more easily than other imaging methods, in some situations your doctor may also order a CT scan or a combination of tests to make an accurate diagnosis. MRI scan can be done without admission to the hospital and is safe.

The downside: The MRI does not give a "totally accurate picture" all the time, and just because there might be abnormal anatomy does not mean that it's the cause of your pain. For instance, studies show that 30 percent of people who have never had back pain also have abnormal findings on the MRI. MRI is also more expensive than a CT scan.

The bottom line: In most cases, you can have the report from an MRI in a day or so, depending on the area to be scanned and the type of report your doctor requested. This tool is considered by most health care professionals to be a very reliable, noninvasive tool for detecting pain-related problems.

Computerized Tomography

Computerized tomography (CT) is used to give a more detailed diagnosis of the internal organs and is especially useful for imaging bones. Computed tomography is a well-known diagnostic study that was used for most complex imaging before MRI became clinically available. CT technique employs ionizing radiation (with or without contrast agents) to create two-dimensional images (slices) of the body. Although many of the uses of CT imaging are now replaced by magnetic resonance imaging (MRI), there is still a place for this test. For instance, CT is especially good for imaging bone; MRI is better, in general, for soft tissue imaging.

With computerized tomography, doctors can make a diagnosis, and then guide surgery and biopsies, target radiation treatment, and drain abscesses.

The procedure: Wearing a hospital gown or robe, you will lie on a flat, narrow table that can turn at different angles, depending on the area of the body to be scanned. The technician will use straps to make sure you are held securely. A leaded apron might be placed over your pelvic area unless those organs are to be scanned. An intravenous contrast dye may be given during the examination to give a clearer picture of internal organs.

An X ray tube located inside a doughnut-shaped machine rotates around your body and emits radiation throughout at different angles. Inside the machine are tiny detectors that calculate the radiation leaving the body and change this into electrical signals. These signals are transferred to a computer, which color-codes them and displays the images on a computer monitor for a radiologist to read.

What you might feel: This procedure has no unusual feelings.

Precautions: If you are allergic to shellfish, let the technician know, as you might have a reaction to the dye.

The upside: Computerized tomography (CT) gives more details of internal organs than an X ray. Using this scan, your doctor may be able to see infections, fractures, and even cancer.

The downside: Like most tests, CT is not perfect. For instance, if you have back pain, this test may suggest you have an abnormal disc in the spine when it is actually normal or at least not causing your pain (called a false positive).

The bottom line: A CT scan does have an acceptable level of radiation exposure, and it can be done on an outpatient basis.

Other Imaging Tests

 • *Bone scans* can detect abnormal areas in all bones of the body, including the spine, and are used in some cases when there is suspicion of infection, fractures, or cancer. Your nuclear medicine team will inject a small amount of radioactive material, which travels through your bloodstream. The radioactivity will collect in the bones, especially in abnormal areas, and is detected by a scanner. While the bone scan does not replace the tests described above, it may add information by eliminating other serious problems. The test is not painful, and the radioactive substance disintegrates.

 • *Myelogram* is a special X ray that requires an injection of dye into the spinal canal through a spinal tap to detect the rupture of a disc or other problems. In a normal myelogram, the dye will fill the spinal canal, as well as the nerve root sheaths, giving a revealing outline for an X ray. In an abnormal myelogram, an absence of that dye occurs in a specific area called a filling defect, and it indicates that the nerve root or spinal cord may be pinched or compressed. This test when combined with a CT scan detects a rupture in more than 90 percent of cases. The myelogram causes some discomfort and has a greater possibility of unwanted side effects, such as painful headache. Most experts now recommend an MRI of the lower spine first. Then, if the diagnosis is not clear, they may perform a myelogram. A CT scan may be combined with a myelogram to improve the accuracy of the diagnosis, especially if a small piece of disc has broken off and is pressing on a nerve away from its root between the vertebrae (off to the side).

● *Discogram* is another study your doctor may use to evaluate the disc. As you lie facedown on the procedure table, the doctor will inject a dye into the disc suspected of being problematic as well as discs they suspect are normal. They may also inject the disc while monitoring the pressure to see if this reproduces your symptoms. The surgeon will use a three-dimensional imaging under radio-television control to find the source of your back pain. Radiographic films are taken, and if the film shows that the dye has leaked out of the disc, your doctor gains more information that the disc may be problematic. This test is often combined with a CT scan for greater accuracy. Within hours, the dye is excreted from the body in the urine.

● *Electromyelogram (EMG) and Nerve Conduction Study* are tests that are used in combination to diagnose sources of pain. An EMG measures the activity of the muscles supplied by the nerves that are being irritated by your ruptured or herniated disc. It is used to help diagnose carpal tunnel syndrome and other nerve or muscle disorders. A nerve conduction study tests the speed of transmission of the nerve signal. In other words, if the nerve is pinched, its ability to transmit a signal is reduced. Abnormal muscle activity and/or slowed nerve conduction may suggest a pinched or irritated nerve from a disc rupture or nerve compression.

● *Bone density test (or bone mineral density or BMD)* is the only guaranteed way to determine bone density and fracture risk for osteoporosis. These tests evaluate the strength of the bones in your body by measuring a small part of one or a few bones. These assessed bones represent the best estimate of fracture risk, although other bones may not have the same bone mineral density. The areas that are most commonly measured are the hip, the lumbar spine (in the lower back), and wrist, the most common sites of fractures due to osteoporosis. Recently, the FDA has approved bone density tests that measure bone density in the middle finger and the heel or shin-bone. These test results show how your bone density compares to that of a normal young woman, as well as to women your age.

Trust Your Doctor

This chapter has discussed the basic tests doctors use to diagnose common types of pain in women. While there are far too many medical tests to discuss all of them in this part of the book, talk openly with your doctor to gain a full understanding before you agree to any test or procedure. For instance, if you suffer with abdominal or pelvic pain, your gynecologist may order an ultra-sound screening or do an endometrial biopsy. Ask questions about what you might expect during the test and if there are any precau-tions you should take. Talk to someone who has had the test to get a patient's perspective. Moreover, make sure the test is necessary in order to make an accurate diagnosis.

No matter what type of pain you have, aggressively work with your doctor to find treatment modalities that resolve it so you can become the master of your pain and reclaim your active life!

CHAPTER TEN

Step 2: Find the Most Effective Medications

The statement "one size doesn't fit all," is true when it comes to medication. For years, doctors have prescribed the same adult dosage of drugs for both men and women. Now we realize that a 5'2", 115-pound woman does not need as much medication as a 6'2", 200-pound man, and such doses may even be toxic for some women. That's why taking the same medication your spouse or father takes may not be a safe bet, and a personal evaluation with an experienced health care professional is of utmost importance.

In my practice, I often resort to rational polypharmacy, or combining multiple medications to achieve effects not attainable by using a single medication. These combinations, or cocktails, occasionally have minor interactions, but the benefits usually clearly outweigh the risks. The prescribing of these medication combinations for chronic pain syndromes remains very much an art and should be individualized, depending on your symptoms and health history.

Because each person responds differently to pain medications, periodic consultations with your doctor to evaluate your medications and your health are necessary to stay pain-free without harboring serious side effects. For now, read the following information to see what successful options you can use to end pain and regain an active life.

MEDICATION ALERT!

Always follow the directions on the medication label, unless your doctor directs otherwise. If you are taking another medication prescribed by a different doctor, check with your pain doctor first to make sure you won't have a drug-drug interaction.

Effective Medications to End Pain

Simple Analgesics

WHAT THEY'RE USED FOR AND HOW THEY WORK   Analgesics, including aspirin and acetaminophen, are used to treat back pain, neck pain, TMJ, carpal tunnel, injuries, headache, PMS, menstrual pain, dental pain, muscle pain, fibromyalgia, osteoarthritis, inflammatory arthritis, and everyday aches and pains.

Aspirin blocks the production of prostaglandins, the chemicals in the body that cause pain, inflammation, and swelling. Acetaminophen elevates the pain threshold, so you perceive less pain.

POTENTIAL SIDE EFFECTS   Aspirin can lead to heartburn, nausea or vomiting, stomach ulcers and gastrointestinal bleeding, and increased clotting time for blood. Acetaminophen is relatively free of side effects. And there are some findings that indicate taking over-the-counter analgesics regularly to prevent pain may actually cause more pain in the end! Overuse of over-the-counter analgesics is widespread; the annual consumption of aspirin alone in this country is measured in the thousands of tons. Unfortunately, when someone with headache takes daily medication for symptom relief, a vicious cycle can occur in which the headache seems to come back or "rebound" as the pain medication wears off—leading people to take pain medication very frequently. If this occurs, you should see your doctor.

Some people cannot take aspirin or nonsteroidal anti-inflammatory drugs (NSAIDs) because an aspirin sensitivity occurs in about 10 to 15 percent of people with asthma and in about 30 to 40 percent of those who have asthma and nasal polyps. Symptoms are itching, rashes, hives, swelling, nasal congestion, and wheezing. Talk to your doctor about alternative therapies for resolving pain if you have this sensitivity.

Aspirin

Aspirin should not be taken in the last three months of pregnancy. Do not take aspirin if it has a strong, vinegarlike odor. It is important to discontinue aspirin use prior to dental procedures and any type of surgery because of the change in clotting times of the blood.

Enteric-coated aspirin is formulated to break down in the intestines instead of the stomach. This helps with some stomach discomfort but does not prevent the possibility of stomach ulcers and bleeding. Enteric-coated products should not be taken within two hours of antacids.

Aspirin should not be taken if you are taking warfarin (Coumadin), heparin, probenecid, quinidine, sulfinpyrazone, methotrexate, or valproic acid.

Acetaminophen

One disadvantage to acetaminophen is that it has a ceiling effect to analgesia, meaning higher doses do not work better. There is also a possibility of liver damage with one very high dose of acetaminophen or a prolonged period of moderately high doses. If you drink more than three alcoholic beverages in a day, liver toxicity may occur at much lower doses if you are taking acetaminophen. In addition, many prescription pain medications contain high doses of acetaminophen, so do not add additional doses of acetaminophen when taking these.

Acetaminophen's drug interactions include alcohol, choestryramine, isoniazid, and phenytoin.

COMMONLY USED ANALGESICS

Brand Name	Generic Name
Advil	ibuprofen
Aleve	naproxen
Anacin	aspirin
Anacin-3	acetaminophen
Anacin Maximum Strength	acetaminophen
Ascriptin, buffered aspirin	aspirin
Bayer	aspirin
Bufferin	buffered aspirin
Excedrin Extra Strength	aspirin plus acetaminophen
Motrin IB	ibuprofen
Norwich	aspirin
Nuprin	ibuprofen
Orudis	ketoprofen
Panex	acetaminophen

Tylenol	acetaminophin
Vanquish	aspirin, plus acetaminophen
Zorprin	12-hour aspirin

Nonsteroidal Anti-inflammatory Drugs (NSAIDs)

WHAT THEY'RE USED FOR AND HOW THEY WORK
Other than aspirin, NSAIDs are the most heavily used drugs in the world. They are commonly used to treat back pain, neck pain, TMJ, carpal tunnel, injuries, headache, PMS, menstrual pain, dental pain, muscle pain, fibromyalgia, osteoarthritis, inflammatory arthritis, and everyday aches and pains. NSAIDs can be taken orally or as injections in the painful site. In some cases, these drugs are compounded by the pharmacist into topical creams, gels, and ointments that are applied directly to the inflamed joint. Applying the medication topically may reduce systemic side effects.

These drugs work as an anti-inflammatory and pain reliever. Like aspirin, NSAIDs block the production of prostaglandins that cause inflammation, pain, and stiffness.

POTENTIAL SIDE EFFECTS   While the pain-relieving effect is excellent with NSAIDs, it does not occur without possible side effects. These drugs may lead to abdominal pain, abnormal liver tests (blood tests), asthma in those allergic to NSAIDs, aggravation of or kidney failure, dizziness, gastritis, heartburn, increased blood pressure, indigestion, intestinal bleeding, anemia, decrease of platelet effect, peptic ulcers, and ringing in the ears.

NSAIDs should be used with caution if you have kidney or liver disease, congestive heart failure, high blood pressure, diabetes, lupus, asthma, or ulcers. Additional monitoring of your dose is necessary if you are taking anticoagulants, cyclosporine, lithium, or methotrexate. If you have aspirin sensitivity use NSAIDs with caution.

COMMONLY USED NONSTEROIDAL ANTI-INFLAMMATORY DRUGS (NSAIDs)

Brand Name	**Generic Name**
Advil	ibuprofen
Aleve	naproxen
Anaprox	naproxen

(continued)

Ansaid	flurbiprofen
Arthrotec	diclofenac plus Misoprostal
Aspirin Products	aspirin
Cataflam	diclofenac
Clinoril	sulindac
Daypro	oxaprozin
Disalcid, Salflex	salsalate
Dolobid	diflunisal
Feldene	piroxicam
Indocin	indomethacin
Lodine	etodolac
Nalfon	fenoprofen
Naprosyn EC	naproxen (enteric-coated)
Naprelan	naproxen delayed release
Naprosyn	naproxen
Oruvail	ketoprofen delayed release
Relafen	nabumetone
Tolectin	tolmetin
Toradol	ketorolac tromethamine
Trilisate	choline magnesium trisalicylate
Voltaren	diclofenac

COX-2 Inhibitors

WHAT THEY'RE USED FOR AND HOW THEY WORK   Cox-2 inhibitors (Super Aspirins) are medications used to treat back and neck pain, TMJ, carpal tunnel, injuries, headache, PMS and menstrual pain, dental pain, muscle pain, fibromyalgia, osteoarthritis, inflammatory arthritis, and everyday aches and pains, among others.

The unwanted actions of prostaglandins cause the pain that bothers most of us, as prostaglandins send messages to trigger inflammation, resulting in pain and swelling. Aspirin and traditional NSAIDs block the prostaglandins, thus blocking inflammation and reducing pain and stiffness. But prostaglandins send a few good messages as well, ones that protect the stomach lining and kidneys. Therefore, by blocking prostaglandins entirely, aspirin and traditional NSAIDs leave us vulnerable to the risk of stomach ulcers, bleeding, and even kidney damage.

About ten years ago, scientists discovered that there were actually two forms of the Cox enzyme cells needed to produce prostaglandins. They realized that the Cox-1 enzyme was very common in normal tissues and helped maintain the normal workings of tissues in the stomach and kidney and other areas, while the Cox-2 form controlled inflammation, mainly in joints and other areas of inflammation in the body. In this breakthrough discovery, scientists realized that the real target to stopping inflammation and pain is the Cox-2 enzyme. The new Cox-2 inhibitors, or Super Aspirins, block this key enzyme, which may possibly result in less inflammation and pain with fewer side effects. While side effects may be less with Cox-2 inhibitors, in clinical trials there were reports of abdominal pain, diarrhea, headache, indigestion, nausea, respiratory infection, and sinus inflammation.

SPECIAL PRECAUTIONS   Use Celebrex with caution after checking with your doctor, if you have sulfa or aspirin allergies. Also, if you have asthma or are taking an anticoagulant medication, use all Cox-2 inhibitors with caution. There is some questionable cardio-vascular risk for those with ischemic heart disease. And while the risk of gastrointestinal bleeding is reduced with Cox-2 inhibitors, it is not totally eliminated.

Possible drug interactions: Ace-inhibitors, diflucan, lasix, lithium, thiazide diuretics. NSAIDs and aspirin should not be taken with Cox-2 inhibitors.

COMMONLY USED COX-2 INHIBITORS

Brand Name	Generic Name
Celebrex	celecoxib
Vioxx	rofecoxib
Bextra	valdecoxib

Corticosteroids

WHAT THEY'RE USED FOR AND HOW THEY WORK   In some situations, corticosteroids are prescribed to treat back pain, neck pain, TMJ, carpal tunnel injuries, headache, muscle pain, osteoarthritis, inflammatory arthritis, and bone pain, among others.

These medications inhibit the production of prostaglandins and leukotrienes, as well as that of certain cytokines, such as interleukin 1. Corticosteroids may be used daily, every other day, in short high dose "bursts," or in tapered dosing.

While the pain relief may be great with corticosteroids, so are the deleterious side effects, including diarrhea or constipation, headache, bone loss, increased or decreased appetite, increased sweating, nervousness, restlessness, difficulty sleeping, upset stomach, "moon" face, and unusual or increased hair on the face or body.

SPECIAL PRECAUTIONS   The greatest concern with these drugs comes with prolonged use, which may lead to problems such as adrenal suppression, fluid and electrolyte disturbances, risk of gastritis, decreased cell-mediated immunity, increased risk of infection, and emotional instability or psychoses. There is the possibility of drug interactions with Rifampin, macrolide antibiotics, Dilantin (Phenytoin), and barbiturates.

COMMONLY USED CORTICOSTEROIDS

Brand Name	Generic Name
Deltasone, Sterapred	prednisone
Medrol	methylprednisolone
Prelone, Orapred	prednisolone
Decadron	dexamethasone

Narcotic Pain Relievers

WHAT THEY'RE USED FOR AND HOW THEY WORK   For moderate to severe pain, narcotic pain relievers (also called opioids) may be prescribed. These drugs are used sometimes to treat back or neck pain, headache, PMS, menstrual pain, dental pain, muscle pain, fibromyalgia, osteoarthritis, inflammatory arthritis, and everyday strains. However, they are often reserved for severe refractory pain that is unresponsive to other treatments.

Opioids work on the central nervous system pain receptors to reduce perception of pain. These narcotic products are available in a wide variety of delivery systems, including patches and liquids, in addition to standard dosage forms.

Narcotic pain relievers may cause serious side effects, such as anxiety, constipation, depression or irritability, dizziness, drowsiness, exaggerated sense of well-being, light-headedness, nausea, and vomiting.

SPECIAL PRECAUTIONS Narcotic pain relievers are potentially addictive, and higher doses may lead to more side effects. If taken for long periods, you may experience withdrawal symptoms if you suddenly stop taking narcotics or dramatically decrease the dose. Some patients are very sensitive to narcotics and become extremely nauseated when taking these drugs. Patients even think they are "allergic" to these products because they become so ill. One product, meperidine, may cause so much nausea that it is combined with promethazine (antinausea agent) in a product called Mepergan Fortis.

COMMONLY USED NARCOTIC PAIN RELIEVERS

Brand Name	*Generic Name*
Darvon	propoxyphene
Darvocet, Wygesic	propoxyphene with acetaminophen
Darvon Compound	propoxyphene with aspirin
Demerol	meperidine
Duragesic	fentanyl
Kadian, MS Contin, Oramorph	morphine
OxyContin, Oxy IR	oxycodone
Stadol (nasal spray)	butorphanol
Talacen	pentazocine with acetaminophen
Talwin NX	pentazocine with naloxone
Tylenol #2, #3, #4, Phenaphen with codeine	codeine with acetaminophen
Tylox, Percocet, Roxicet, Endocet	oxycodone with acetaminophen
Vicodin, Lortab, Lorcet, Norco	hydrocodone with acetaminophen
Vicoprofen	hydrocodone with ibuprofen

Muscle Relaxants

WHAT THEY'RE USED FOR AND HOW THEY WORK Muscle relaxants are often used to treat moderate to severe TMJ, headache, muscle pain, fibromyalgia, and everyday sprains and strains.

These pain-relieving medications work in the central nervous system to "relax" skeletal muscles.

With muscle relaxants, you may experience dry mouth, dizziness, drowsiness, blurred vision, clumsiness, unsteadiness, and a change in the color of your urine. These medications may increase likelihood of seizures, and older adults sometimes experience confusion and hallucinations.

SPECIAL PRECAUTIONS   Muscle relaxants may negatively interact with other drugs such as MAO inhibitors, barbiturates, guanethidine, Ultram (tramadol), central nervous system depressants, alcohol, and tricyclic antidepressants. Use caution if you take any of these, and talk to your doctor before using narcotic medications with muscle relaxants.

COMMONLY USED MUSCLE RELAXANTS

Brand Name	Generic Name
Flexeril	cyclobenzaprine
Lioresal	baclofen
Norflex	orphenadrine citrate
Parafon	chlorzoxazone
Robaxin	methocarbamol
Skelaxin	metaxalone
Soma	carisoprodol
Zanaflex	tizanidine

Nonnarcotic Analgesics

WHAT THEY'RE USED FOR AND HOW THEY WORK   Nonnarcotic analgesics are commonly used to treat moderate to moderately severe pain, such as back and neck pain, dental pain, injuries, and headache.

The nonnarcotic medication acts centrally in the brain to modulate the sensation of pain, yet it has no anti-inflammatory effect.

With nonnarcotic medications, you may also experience agitation, anxiety, bloating, gas, constipation, convulsive movements, diarrhea, dizziness, drowsiness, dry mouth, feeling of elation, hallucinations, headache, indigestion, itching, nausea, nervousness, sweating, tremor, vomiting, and weakness.

Special Precautions   Watch for drug interactions if you are taking the following: carbamazepine, cyclobenzaprine, MAO inhibitors, SSRIs, tricyclic antidepressants, Thorazine, Stelazine, promethazine, quinidine, narcotic pain relievers, sleeping medications (Halcion, Dalmane, Restoril) and other benzodiazepines (Valium, Xanax, and Klonopin).

There is still a chance of dependence with nonnarcotic medications, especially in those patients who have had a dependence problem before. There is a possibility of withdrawal symptoms when discontinuing Ultram. A gradual decrease will prevent this from being a major problem.

Avoid alcohol when taking nonnarcotic medications. Large doses of this drug, or the combination with various other drugs, may cause seizures. You should also avoid these medications (e.g. tramadol) if you are taking MAO inhibitors.

Commonly Used Nonnarcotic Analgesics

Brand Name	**Generic Name**
Ultracet	tramadol plus acetaminophen
Ultram	tramadol

Anticonvulsants

What They're Used For and How They Work   Anticonvulsants are often used to treat TMJ, nerve pain, migraines, and some types of cancer pain.

Anticonvulsants may work by decreasing substance P activity and stabilizing neuronal activity in the brain nerves at sufficiently high doses.

Some common side effects with certain anticonvulsants include dizziness, somnolence, weight gain, tremor, and gum problems. Topamax has been found to cause weight loss.

Special Precautions   Because each of the anticonvulsants appears to have a different mechanism of action, if one fails, talk to your doctor about trying another. Depakote has been shown to be most effective in patients with severe migraines without auras.

COMMONLY USED ANTICONVULSANTS

Brand Names	Generic Names
Depakote	diralproex sodium
Dilantin	phenytoin
Gabitril	tiagabine
Lamictal	lamotrigine
Neurontin	gabapentin
Tegretol	carbamazepine
Topamax	topiramate
Trileptal	oxcarbazepine
Zonegran	zonisamide

Tricyclic Antidepressants

WHAT THEY'RE USED FOR AND HOW THEY WORK   Tricyclic antidepressants are often used in combination with other medications to treat back pain, neck pain, chronic pelvic pain, migraine and headache pain, fibromyalgia, and other types of chronic pain.

These antidepressants help to improve sleep, which may lead to an increase in endorphins, the body's natural painkiller. They also increase levels of serotonin and norepinephrine in the brain. Patients with chronic pain often have decreased levels of these calming neurotransmitters.

Tricyclic antidepressants may cause drowsiness, dizziness, dry mouth, dry eyes, and constipation.

SPECIAL PRECAUTIONS   These medications may interact with MAO inhibitors, cimetidine, and other central nervous system depressants.

COMMONLY USED TRICYCLIC ANTIDEPRESSANTS

Name Brand	Generic Brand
Elavil	amitriptyline
Desyrel	trazodone
Norpramin	desipramine
Pamelor	nortriptyline
Sinequan	doxepin
Tofranil	imipramine

Selective Serotonin Reuptake Inhibitors (SSRIs)

WHAT THEY'RE USED FOR AND HOW THEY WORK
SSRIs are commonly used to treat back pain, neck pain, chronic pelvic pain, migraines, fibromyalgia, PMS, menstrual pain, fibromyalgia, and osteoarthritis.

By blocking the reuptake of serotonin, SSRIs allow more serotonin to travel from neuron to neuron, resulting in improved symptoms.

With SSRIs, you may feel side effects such as tremors, drowsiness, sweating, nervousness, sexual side effects, dry mouth, insomnia, headache, nausea, diarrhea, and loss of interest in eating.

SPECIAL PRECAUTIONS   SSRIs may interact negatively with drugs such as phenytoin, carbamazepine, anti-psychotics, benzodiazepines, tryptophan, MAO inhibitors, warfarin, and thioridazine. Talk with your doctor before taking SSRIs if you are also taking these medications.

COMMONLY USED SELECTIVE SEROTONIN REUPTAKE INHIBITORS	
Brand Name	**Generic Name**
Celexa	citalopram
Paxil	paroxetine
Prozac	fluoxetine
Luvox	fluvoxamine
Zoloft	sertraline

Benzodiazepines

WHAT THEY'RE USED FOR AND HOW THEY WORK   Benzodiazepines are often used to treat associated anxiety that accompanies chronic pain. These medications also have some muscle relaxant properties.

These medications act to depress the central nervous system and result in sedation, hypnosis, skeletal muscle relaxation, anticonvulsant activity, and sometimes coma in large doses.

With benzodiazepines, you may experience drowsiness, fatigue, light-headedness, and loss of muscle coordination.

SPECIAL PRECAUTIONS   Watch for drug-drug interactions if you are also taking cimetidine, erythromycin, disulfiram, phenytoin, CNS depressants, or digoxin. Benzodiazepines may also interfere with your ability to function because of negative effects on cognition. In some cases, these drugs can exacerbate depression, and many patients with chronic pain already have increased problems with depression. Benzodiazepines are psychologically and physically addictive.

COMMONLY USED BENZODIAZEPINES

Name Brand	Generic Brand
Ativan	lorazepam
Klonopin	clonazepam
Valium	diazepam
Xanax	alprazolam

Lidocaine

WHAT IT'S USED FOR AND HOW IT WORKS   Lidocaine patches are used for many types of pain, including diabetic neuropathy, post-herpetic neuralgia, and sometimes even chronic low back pain. Lidocaine has also been used in nasal drops to provide effective relief for migraine sufferers. One case report suggests that taking it during the aura phase may prevent the development of a full-blown migraine. Side effects of nasal drops are unpleasant taste, burning sensation, and facial numbness. Often the headache will rebound, requiring a second drug.

Lidocaine blocks conduction of impulses and stabilizes neuronal membranes. It acts as an anesthetic, an agent that reduces sensation or numbs.

POTENTIAL SIDE EFFECTS   No systemic effects have been reported. Side effects are limited to treatment area irritation. The area could become red, swollen or there could be an experience of abnormal sensation.

Migraine Treatments

Triptans

WHAT THEY'RE USED FOR AND HOW THEY WORK   Triptans are effective in treating acute migraine headaches. These serotonin agonists work by imitating serotonin and stimulating receptors in the brain, resulting in vasoconstriction and decreased pain message transmission.

With triptans, you may have mild, transient elevation of blood pressure, tingling, sensation of warmth, dizziness, flushing, drowsiness, chest pain, neck/throat/jaw pain, weakness, stomach upset, and nausea.

SPECIAL PRECAUTIONS   Triptans can interact negatively with certain drugs, including SSRIs and MAO inhibitors. Do not take triptans if you are pregnant, or have uncontrolled diabetes, hypertension, or coronary artery disease. Rebound migraines occur in 20 to 40 percent of patients using these drugs. These rebound headaches generally respond to a second dose of drug.

Imitrex is available in injectible, nasal spray, and oral dosage forms. The nasal spray is absorbed very quickly and brings relief in as little as 15 minutes. The spray may leave a bad taste and tends to be less effective if you have nasal congestion. Injectible Imitrex works the fastest, but this type is inconvenient and causes pain at the injection site. Maxalt MLT is a product that dissolves instantly on the tongue. This is useful when the migraine is causing nausea, as there is no need to drink liquids with the tablet.

There is increasing evidence that overuse of these products can exacerbate migraines and recommended dosage is no more than twice a week.

COMMONLY USED TRIPTANS

Brand Names	Generic Names
Axert	almotriptan
Amerge	naratriptan
Frova	frovatriptan
Imitrex	sumatriptan
Maxalt	rizatriptan
Zomig	zolmitriptan

Combination Treatments

There are other effective products for treating acute migraine, including a combination medication consisting of caffeine, butalbital, and analgesic. With this product, the caffeine works as a vasoconstrictor, while butalbital is a barbituate, and acetaminophen and aspirin are simple analgesics (pain relievers).

With this combination product, you may experience abdominal pain, dizziness, drowsiness, intoxicated feeling, light-headedness, nausea, sedation, shortness of breath, and vomiting.

COMMONLY USED COMBINATION PRODUCTS	
Brand Name	**Generic Name**
Esgic, Fioricet	acetaminophen, butalbital, and caffeine
Excedrin Migraine	acetaminophen, aspirin, and caffeine
Fiorinal	aspirin, butalbital, and caffeine
Fiorinal with Codeine	aspirin, butalbital, caffeine, and codeine
Fiorcet with Codeine	butalbital and acetaminophen, caffeine, and codeine
Phrenilin	butalbital and acetaminophen

Serotonin Antagonist

Serotonin antagonists, such as Sansert (methysergide), are sometimes used to prevent or reduce the intensity and frequency of vascular headaches, but not to treat acute headache pain. Along with the pain relief, you may experience nausea, muscle cramps, and abdominal pain. Some people also have weight gain with serotonin antagonists. And this drug cannot be taken by patients with coronary artery disease, peripheral vascular disease, and phlebitis, or cellulitis.

Ergotamines

WHAT THEY'RE USED FOR AND HOW THEY WORK Ergotamines are used to abort or prevent migraine or cluster headaches. Ergotamine tartrate and dihydroergotamine mesylate are potent vasoconstrictors and are believed to bind to serotonin receptors, causing vasoconstriction.

You may experience nausea, abdominal pain, mental disturbances, dizziness, tingling sensations, muscle cramps, and chest pain.

SPECIAL PRECAUTIONS   Ergotamines should not be used if you have hypertension or ischemic heart disease. It is important that ergotamines not be taken within 24 hours of the triptans, such as Imitrex or Sansert (methysergide).

Rebound headaches are very common with ergotamine products. These drugs seem to be helpful in prevention of "predictable" migraine attacks, such as those that occur every month around menstruation.

People who have taken ergotamine for long periods are at higher risk for severe dependency, and withdrawal may require hospitalization.

COMMONLY USED ERGOTAMINES	
Brand Name	**Generic Name**
Cafergot, Wigraine, Ergaf	ergotamine and caffeine
DHE-45, Migranal	dihydroergotamine mesylate

Migraine Propylaxis

There are several drugs, including beta blockers and calcium channel blockers, that are now being used to prevent migraines altogether. These products are generally used in patients that experience two or more migraines per month.

Beta blockers stabilize blood vessels, limiting dilation, but can also have side effects such as fatigue, drowsiness, lethargy, and depression. It's not fully understood how calcium channel blockers work, but it is believed they react with 5HT-1 serotonin receptors. These medications have side effects such as dizziness, swelling, nausea, and headache and should not be used by those with arrthythmias and congestive heart failure. These drugs can cause severe headaches in some patients, which limits their use for prevention of migraine headache.

Other Products Being Investigated for Migraine Relief

- Bromocriptine (Parlodel), an ergot derivative, may be effective against menstrual migraines. While Parlodel seems to work best when taken continuously, the side effects, including lightheadedness and nausea, are often uncomfortable. Parlodel does not seem effective in patients taking oral contraceptives and hormone replacement therapy, and there have been reports of high blood pressure, seizure, and strokes in some taking this drug. Parlodel may also be used to treat amenorrhea and painful breast conditions.

● Ganoxolone (a drug known as an epalon) is an anti-inflammatory, steroidlike drug that affects nerve cells. In clinical trials, ganoxolone produced pain relief in four hours in 87 percent of patients.

● Haloperidol (Haldol), a drug normally given for psychosis, has been found to successfully treat migraine headaches when given in injection form.

NEW DRUG DELIVERY SYSTEMS

Getting medications to the exact site of pain is not easy. Two new drug delivery systems may help to change that. In one system, a special molecule called an axonal transport facilitator carries the drug to the site of the pain and drops it off. This injection can be used at specific sites for pain or injected into muscles, resulting in pain control with fewer side effects. The vaginal ring may be used for medication delivery in women. A ring is currently available for estradiol delivery (Estring), and the FDA has approved for release the contraceptive product (Nuvaring).

Drugs for Reproductive Difficulties

Oral Contraceptives

WHAT THEY'RE USED FOR AND HOW THEY WORK   Oral contraceptives are frequently used to treat endometriosis and dysmenorrhea (menstrual cramps). Oral contraceptives give hormone regulation, as well as decreasing menstrual flow and duration of menstruation. Along with the control of hormonal pain, you may also experience irregular bleeding, mood swings, bloating, headache, and weight gain.

SPECIAL PRECAUTIONS   Oral contraceptives have been known to cause serious life-threatening problems, including stroke, blood clots, and heart attacks, especially in women who are cigarette smokers. These medications should not be used by smokers and women with certain types of cancer and/or a previous history of blood clots.

Injectible Contraceptives

WHAT THEY'RE USED FOR AND HOW THEY WORK   In some cases, injectible contraceptives, such as Depo-Provera (progesterone), are used to treat endometriosis. The injectible contraceptives give a continuous supply of progesterone, which generally stops the menstrual cycle completely.

These medications can increase bleeding in some women. You may also experience weight gain, depression, and other side effects common with oral contraceptives.

SPECIAL PRECAUTIONS   Because this medication is injected, it is not reversible and is effective for three months.

Gonadotropin-Releasing Hormone Agonists

WHAT THEY'RE USED FOR AND HOW THEY WORK Gonadotropin-releasing hormone agonists are commonly used to treat endometriosis. These medications work on the pituitary gland to deplete it of all gonadotropins, creating drug-induced ovarian failure, with symptoms of menopause. With this treatment, areas of endometriosis can stabilize, and pain is reduced.

The side effects of these drugs are usually uncomfortable and include non-menstrual vaginal bleeding, cessation of menstruation, hot flashes, headaches, vaginal dryness, acne, reduction in breast size, bone density loss, and irritation at administration site.

SPECIAL PRECAUTIONS   Over a period of three to six months, these medications cause a reversible medical menopause with subsequent hot flashes and reduced bone density.

COMMONLY USED GONADOTROPIN-RELEASING HORMONE AGONISTS

Brand Name	Generic Name
Lupron	leuprolide acetate
Synarel	nafarelin acetate
Zoladex	goserelin acetate implant

Disease-Modifying Anti-Rheumatic Drugs

The slow-acting, or disease-modifying, medicines are added when rheumatoid arthritis pain and swelling remain a problem even after using other anti-inflammatory medications such as Super Aspirin. In the past, these medications were used after deformities began, often years after the rheumatoid arthritis started. Now they are used much earlier, as soon as it is apparent that the arthritis is not being controlled or at least as soon as permanent changes are seen on X rays.

Methotrexate

Methotrexate (Rheumatrex tablets and injectable methotrexate) is the most popular of the slow-acting medicines to try to stop the progress of rheumatoid arthritis. Studies show that more than 80 percent of rheumatoid patients respond with reduced pain and swelling. In some cases, methotrexate may completely control the symptoms. This medication also delays the progressive bone destruction associated with rheumatoid arthritis. Some new findings indicate that patients who take methotrexate have a 70 percent reduction in cardiovascular mortality and 60 percent lower risk of death overall.

Methotrexate may be combined with other traditional NSAIDs for a better effect. The most common side effect is nausea, which usually occurs within one day of taking the weekly dose of methotrexate. If the nausea is too bothersome, the methotrexate may be given by injection in a muscle, which can diminish the nausea. Mild side effects, such as mouth sores, may be controlled by taking a folic acid supplement. Abnormal liver blood tests, abnormal blood counts, and lung reactions with pneumonia are uncommon but can occur, so regular blood tests and checkups are important.

Azulfidine

Azulfidine (sulfasalazine) is another slow-acting medicine available for the treatment of rheumatoid arthritis that does not respond to anti-inflammatory drugs. This tablet is usually well tolerated and has about a 70 percent chance of decreasing joint pain and stiffness. The improvement may begin four to twelve weeks after starting the medicine. Some studies show that it may slow the progress of arthritis.

The most common side effects are usually mild and include loss of appetite, headache, nausea, and upset stomach. Azulfidine occasionally causes abnormal blood tests (including liver tests), anemia, low white blood cell count, or other blood abnormality. If you try Azulfidine, your doctor will schedule you for regular blood tests.

Plaquenil

Plaquenil (hydroxychloroquine) may be the slow-acting medication with the fewest side effects. The tablet can give relief of joint pain and stiffness and may be used along with other pain medications, such as NSAIDs or methotrexate, to improve the effect. You will need an eye examination once or twice each year to watch for side effects in the retina of the eye, which are extremely rare.

Gold Capsules and Injections

Gold medications have been used for many years, because they effectively relieve the painful symptoms and may slow or stop the progress of rheumatoid arthritis. The capsules (Ridaura) are convenient but have a lower response rate than gold injections. The most common side effect of Ridaura is diarrhea, which happens in 30 percent of patients but then ceases without stopping the medications.

Gold injections (Myochrysine, Solganol) are given in the hip muscle and are usually well tolerated. About 70 to 75 percent of patients respond with decreased pain and swelling. The most common side effects are rash or mouth sores. Regular blood counts and urinalysis are needed with all gold medications for safety to check for side effects on the bone marrow and kidney.

Biological Response Modifiers

WHAT THEY'RE USED FOR AND HOW THEY WORK   Biological response modifiers are commonly used for moderate to severe rheumatoid arthritis. Enbrel and Remicade block the action of tumor necrosis factor (a naturally occuring protein responsible for much of the joint inflammation that plagues patients with rheumatoid arthritis). Arava works by blocking an enzyme called dihydroorotate dehydrogenase (DHODH), which slows down the lymphocytes, white blood cells that trigger inflammation involved in the process that leads to the disease, and subsequently slows the progression of the disease. Kineret is an interleukin-1 receptor antagonist. Interleukin-1 has been shown to be a contributor to the rheumatoid arthritis disease process.

Some possible side effects of these medications include abdominal pain, cough, dizziness, headache, indigestion, infection, injection site reactions, nausea, rash, respiratory problems, sore throat, vomiting, and weakness.

SPECIAL PRECAUTIONS   TNF (tumor necrosis factor) produces inflammation and joint damage in the body, but it also plays a major role in the immune system. Blocking the action of TNF may lower your resistance to infection. In fact, an increase in tuberculosis has been seen in patients taking these medications (TB testing is strongly recommended). Arava has been reported to cause hepatic toxicity, cirrhosis, liver failure, and death. However, it is possible that these were cases of patients poorly monitored while taking this drug.

COMMONLY USED BIOLOGICAL RESPONSE MODIFIERS

Name Brand	Generic Brand
Arava	leflunomide
Enbrel	etanercept
Kineret	anakinra
Remicade	infliximab

DRUG SAFETY

Go to www.ismp.org (The Institute of Safe Medicine Practices) to see if your drug will work with other medicines you are taking.

The Future of Pain Relief

Out on the horizon are multiple new medications that are being evaluated for the treatment of pain. One promising agent, which may prove to be useful in the future, is tropisetron, a 5-HT3-serotonin antagonist. The effect of the 5-HT3-serotonin antagonists is primarily to limit the release of substance P, which acts as a mediator of pain and inflammation. In pilot studies, European researchers found that patients with inflammatory rheumatic diseases, soft-tissue diseases, chronic low back pain, and cervical pain experienced an improvement in pain and decreased inflammation with injections of tropisetron. These results imply that tropisetron could someday supplement or replace traditional therapies in those with pain-related syndromes.

Always Talk to Your Doctor

Now that you know about the most commonly used medications for women's pain, call your doctor. Because of limited space, I have not included every medication that may work to help resolve pain. So make sure your doctor gives you detailed information on any pre-scribed drug therapy, including what it is used for, how it's taken, possible side effects, and special precautions, if any. Bring to the doctor a list of the medications—including dosages—that you are taking, and bring any dietary supplements you are taking with you to the visit.

It's imperative that you don't self-prescribe any of the medications I've discussed without consulting with your physician. Even seemingly "safe" medications can have toxic effects if you are not careful, and your doctor is trained to guide you.

CHAPTER ELEVEN

Step 3: Try a Combination of Natural Cures

In chapters 4 through 8, I explained the most common types of pain that women experience, giving you the specific modalities that help to treat the pain. Once you've confirmed the type of pain with your doctor and have evaluated the best medications to treat this, as discussed in Steps 1 and 2, look at how natural therapies work and how you can incorporate these into your lifestyle. The following are some of the most common natural therapies women can use to end pain.

Hydrotherapy

The use of hydrotherapy goes back to ancient Greece, when all forms of water—from ice to steam—were used to promote healing and well-being. In the eighteenth and early nineteenth century, hydrotherapy became a popular form of treatment with the invention of the sponge bath, the wet sheet pack, and the spa. (Wet sheet packing involved wrapping the patient in wet sheets for varying periods with the intent of chilling, then over-heating, the body to get rid of toxins.)

Hydrotherapy works by stimulating your body's own healing force. For instance, cold compresses reduce swelling by constricting blood vessels, helping to control minor internal bleeding. Conversely, warm, moist compresses on the painful area dilate blood vessels, which in turn lowers blood pressure and increases the flow of blood, oxygen and nutrients, and speeds the elimination of toxins.

Hydrotherapy works well for almost all types of pain. When the pain first starts to flare, it's important to treat it *immediately* with compresses of either ice or heat on the painful site—whichever brings you the most relief. For instance, ice can reduce the pain of an injury such as a sprain or strain if used at least ten minutes *each waking hour* for the first seventy-eight hours after injury. Moist heat may give relief to chronic pain like an arthritic hip or monthly menstrual cramps. You may use a moist heating pad; a warm, damp towel; or a hydrocollator pack. You can also stand or sit on a stool in the shower and let warm water hit the painful area on your body.

When you use moist heat to decrease pain and swelling, use it twice a day or more, at least twenty minutes each time. You may want to alternate the ice compresses with the moist heat for optimal benefit. You may use moist heat for a few minutes just before and after stretching or resistance or aerobic exercise to make it less painful and more effective.

USE RICE FOR ACUTE INJURIES

If your pain stems from a muscle injury, treat it immediately with RICE: Rest, Ice, Compression, and Elevation. Rest the injured body part, and then apply ice (an ice pack or pack of frozen vegetables or fruit) for twenty minutes on, then twenty minutes off. Add compression with a firm elastic bandage. Elevate the injured part to keep swelling minimal.

Balneotherapy

Many of my patients also find long-lasting relief with balneotherapy, or the use of hot baths or spas to alleviate pain. This centuries-old therapy helps to increase muscle relaxation, boost blood supply to the site, and relieve rigidity and spasms in the muscles of patients with fibromyalgia, arthritis, back pain, menstrual discomfort, and most other types of pain. Epsom salts or bicarbonate of soda can be added to therapeutic warm baths to assist in pain relief and detoxification.

If you suffer with abdominal or menstrual cramps or pelvic pain, a sitz bath—a warm water bath that covers the lower abdomen, hips, and buttocks—can sometimes give almost instant relief. Some women add Epsom salts to the warm sitz bath to increase healing.

A Jacuzzi is another excellent form of balneotherapy. (Caution: Avoid hot tubs or spas if you have diabetes, high blood pressure, cardiovascular disease, or are pregnant.)

Heating Pad

While moist heat helps most types of pain, according to a study published in the March 2001 issue of the *Journal of Obstetrics and Gynecology*, curling up with a heating pad may help ease menstrual cramps as much as ibuprofen, an over-the-counter nonsteroidal anti-inflammatory drug (NSAID). Researchers are unsure as to the pain-reducing mechanism of heat, but they do know that heat is a vasodilator that reduces constriction of blood vessels and improves blood flow to the uterus. Heat may alter a woman's threshold for pain in a similar way to placebo or relax the uterus by reducing the activity of the digestive tract. Women in the study who used both heat and ibuprofen reported relief after 90 minutes; women who used ibuprofen without heat felt relief nearly 3 hours later. If hot water bottles and electric heating pads are inconvenient to use, there are new "heat patches" you can apply to your skin and wear for eight hours. The patches allow complete mobility with continuous constant heat.

Castor Oil Pack

Castor oil has been used for centuries to boost healing by reducing pain and inflammation. To make a castor oil pack, pour some castor oil onto a dry cloth until the cloth is wet but not dripping. Place the cloth on the painful area, put a plastic covering over the wet oiled cloth, and then put a heating pad or hot water bottle on top. Use this daily for twenty minutes or until the pain subsides.

Natural Supplements

By definition, natural supplements contain substances like vitamins, herbs, minerals, and amino acids. Some of these supplements inhibit the system's inflammatory cytokines, which otherwise would become elevated in chronic pain conditions. Others block the pain-causing prostaglandins and leukotrienes, chemicals in the body that cause inflammation. There are natural therapies that appear to boost endorphins, the body's natural opioids that relieve pain; others help heal an exhausted immune system and repair damaged tissue.

As I've learned more about natural therapies, I realize that some alternative therapies are viable treatment for women with chronic pain. While these therapies have not been tested as rigorously as pharmaceuticals, that does not mean that all are sham. Most physicians are aware of medications that have been well tested yet still have deleterious side effects. A good Web site that keeps consumers informed about dietary supplements that may be unsafe or recalled is www.fda.gov/medwatch/safety.htm. Check this site periodically to make sure you are taking safe supplements. Also, be sure and let your doctors know that you are taking dietary supplements as they may have unrecognized side effects or interact with one of your medications.

I've found that some natural therapies may work well for one patient, yet do nothing for another patient. In addition, most alternative treatments work best in conjunction with prescribed medical therapies. That's why talking openly with your doctor before you take any unproven treatment will help you get the best of both worlds and find the safest treatments that work for you.

RED FLAG!

Sometimes a supplement or herb may counteract the effects of your prescription medication, leaving your doctor baffled when the medicine is ineffective, and your pain is worse. Sometimes a natural therapy may cause liver damage or other serious side effects. Use caution with any unproven treatment. Remember, just because something is natural does not mean that it is always safe. As Socrates realized too late, hemlock, a poisonous plant, is very natural—but deadly!

Herbal Remedies to Ease Pain

The one problem with natural dietary supplements—even though some may work—is that you are never sure what you are really getting when you make the purchase. Because dietary supplements are considered "food items" and are not regulated by the Food and

Drug Administration, manufacturers are not held accountable for claims they make or for what they grind up and sell to consumers.

When choosing herbs, look for the ones labeled "standardized." This means the manufacturer measured the amount of key ingredients in the herbal batch. Since plants can vary greatly in their potency, and there is no government regulation for ingredients in herbal remedies, the chances are greater that you will get what you pay for in a "standardized brand." Also, buy herbs made by a reputable manufacturer rather than an off-brand that may be cheaper. Some of the known brands include General Nutrition, Natrol, Sundown, Your Life, Mother Nature, and Nature's Bounty, among others. You might ask your pharmacist to recommend a reputable brand.

If you decide to take any of the following herbal supplements, play it safe, and talk to your doctor, pharmacist or a certified nutritionist about side effects. Herbal therapies are not recommended for pregnant women, children, the elderly, or those with compromised immune systems. In addition, some herbs have sedative or blood-thinning qualities, which may dangerously interact with NSAIDs or other pain medications. Others may cause gastrointestinal upset if taken in large doses. For example, ginkgo biloba may cause nausea, diarrhea, stomach upset, and vomiting if taken in larger doses and may reduce clotting time. Anyone taking coumadin should not take this herb. If you are taking drugs with a narrow therapeutic index such as cyclosporine, digoxin, hypoglycemic agents, lithium, phenytoin, procainamide, theophylline, tricyclic antidepressants, and warfarin, you should avoid herbal products altogether. In addition, St. John's wort, which is taken by many for the treatment of depression, may cause serious herb-drug reactions, particularly if taken with SSRI agents.

Ask your doctor about the following herbs, and if you decide to use herbal therapy, follow the package directions for appropriate dosage.

Boswellia (*Boswellia serrata*). Inhibits leukotrienes, pro-inflammatory chemicals in the body, and improves the blood supply to joint tissues. Some women with arthritis find that boswellia reduces joint swelling and morning stiffness, helps to increase mobility, and reduces arthritic pain.
- Available as tincture, dried leaves and stems, or capsules.
- Side effects are uncommon but may include nausea, diarrhea, and skin rash.

Burdock root *(Arctium lappa).* Promotes healthy kidney function and helps prevent water retention. Burdock is said to help ease arthritis and rheumatism pain and swelling.
- Available as dried powder, tincture, and pieces of root. Follow package directions.
- Should not be used by children or pregnant women as it can stimulate the uterus.

Capsicum (cayenne, hot pepper) *(Capsicum species).* Relieves migraine or tension headaches when taken internally and helps to ease pain of arthritis. Used as a cream or ointment, capsaicin is effective in preventing muscle aches, back or neck pain, arthritis pain, and sprains.
- Available as dried herb, supplements, and ointments.
- Avoid contact with eyes, genitals, or open wounds, and before using topically, do a skin test for sensitivity. If taken orally in large doses, capsicum may cause stomach upset, vomiting, and diarrhea.

Devil's claw *(Harpagophytum procumbens).* Eases pain and stiffness of arthritis, back pain, and menstrual cramps when used as an herbal replacement for nonsteroid anti-inflammatory drugs (NSAIDs).
- Available as capsules, dried root in tea, tincture, or extract.
- There appears to be no serious risk of side effects, although some have reported mild gastrointestinal upset.

Feverfew *(Tanacetum parthenium L).* Reduces inflammation as well as prostaglandins, the chemical compounds in the body that cause pain and swelling. Feverfew's actions resemble those of aspirin, and it might therefore prove useful in treating arthritis. Canada's Health Protection Branch recognizes feverfew as a nonprescription drug for preventing migraines.
- Available as dried leaf, tablets, or capsules.
- Anyone with a clotting disorder should consult a physician before taking feverfew.

Ginger *(Zingiber officinale).* Reduces inflammation and symptoms of osteoarthritis in clinical studies. In findings published in the November 2001 issue of *Arthritis and Rheumatism*, 63 percent of the patients with osteoarthritis of the knee who took ginger reported reduced pain in the knee while standing and less pain after walking 50 feet. Ginger has also been used to treat migraine headache.

- Available as powdered or fresh root, tincture, dried leaves and stems, capsule, or as a spice to use in cooking.
- May cause gastrointestinal discomfort.

Hawthorn (*Crataegus oxyacantha*).   Strengthens tissues and supports healing. Hawthorn is high in flavonoids, especially anthocyanidins and proanthocyanidins, which help strengthen connective tissue.

- Available as dried berries for tea and tincture.
- There seem to be no known toxicity problems.

Meadowsweet (*Filipendula ulmaria*).   Eases pain of arthritis or other inflammatory diseases because it has aspirinlike chemicals.

- Available in dried leaves and root, and extract.
- Because of the aspirinlike quality, do not take meadowsweet if you have a blood disorder or are taking any nonsteroidal anti-inflammatory medications (NSAIDs).

Nettle (*Urtica dioica*).   Contains a variety of natural chemicals that may help lower pain, swelling, and inflammation. These chemicals also help slow the actions of many enzymes that trigger inflammation. Nettle leaf has been used for years in Germany as a safe treatment of arthritis. In a study published in the May 2000 issue of the *Journal of the Royal Society of Medicine*, researchers applied stinging nettle leaves to the hands of twenty-seven arthritis sufferers. After one week, they found that stinging nettles not only significantly reduced pain, but also that the level of that pain stayed lower through most of the treatment. They concluded that nettles contain serotonin and histamine, both neurotransmitters that affect pain perception and transmission at the nerve endings.

- Available as tincture, dried leaves and stems, or in capsules.
- Excessive amounts of nettle may cause stomach irritation, constipation, or burning skin. If you are allergic to pollen, avoid nettle.

Turmeric (*Curcuma longa*).   Protects the body against the ravages of free radicals, naturally occurring toxic substances. Turmeric, native to southern Asia, is a member of the ginger family and has a potent anti-inflammatory compound, curcumin. Use turmeric as spice on foods, mixed in hot tea or warm milk, or in capsules.

- Available as a spice, leaves, dried root, essential oil, and capsules.
- Side effects may include gastrointestinal upset.

White willow bark (*Salix alba*).   Has an analgesic effect and is tagged the "first nonsteroidal anti-inflammatory drug (NSAID)." White willow bark was used in ancient China as early as 500 B.C. In a study published in the *British Journal of Rheumatology*, researchers compared the effectiveness of willow bark (Assalix) with a Cox-2 inhibitor. Both groups reported a decrease in pain. Researchers concluded that there was no significant difference in effectiveness between the two treatments at the doses chosen, but treatment with white willow bark was about 40 percent less expensive.

- Available as powdered bark, supplements, and decoction.
- If you are allergic to aspirin and/or other NSAIDs, avoid taking willow bark.

Botanicals for Menstrual Cramps and Pelvic Congestion

Numerous botanical (plant) medicines have been used throughout history specifically to treat painful menstruation. In Europe, women rely on yarrow (*Achillea millefolium*) in hot tea or sitz baths to help ease cramping. Ginger, an herb used for menstrual pain in China, Japan, and India, is highly valued particularly because of its soothing, antispasmodic properties.

While not fully substantiated by science, some of the following herbal therapies appear to have some therapeutic influence in the body:

Dong Quai (*Angelica sinensis*).   Used to relieve menstrual discomfort, boost production of red blood cells, and treat weakness and fatigue.

- Available as dried herb, tablets, capsules, or tincture. Follow package directions.
- Angelica should not be used by pregnant women and can cause fever and excessive menstrual bleeding in some women.

Ginger root (*Zingiber officinale*).   Used to ease nausea and gastrointestinal discomfort associated with menstruation.

- Available as dried root, powder, capsules or tablets, dried herb for tea, and as spice to be used in cooking and baking.
- Ginger root can cause heartburn.

Vitex Chaste tree (*Vitex agnus-castus*).   Taken for menstrual disorders by women since Greco-Roman times and approved in Germany for treating menstrual disorders, PMS, and painful breasts. Extract of vitex helps regulate menstrual cycle, causing symptoms to lessen.

- Available as capsules and liquid extract.
- Side effects include skin rash, itching, and gastrointestinal upset.

Evening primrose (*Oenothera biennis*).   Used to reduce inflammation. Evening primrose oil contains essential fatty acids such as gamma linolenic acid (GLA), an important component of cellular structures in the body. GLA can be converted to a compound called prostaglandin E-1, which helps to decrease blood clotting and inflammation.

- Available as seed, oil, bark, leaves, and capsules.
- Side effects include headache, nausea, and diarrhea.

Red clover (*Trifolium pratense*).   Used to ease the pain of menstrual cramps. Red clover, said to have a higher isoflavone level than soy, is used as a muscle relaxer.

- Available as dried flowers, tincture, and capsules.
- Recognized as generally safe by the FDA.

Energizing Herbal Therapies

If chronic pain has left you fatigued and without motivation, the following herbal therapies may energize you.

Asian ginseng (*Panax ginseng*).   Boosts the immune response by increasing the number of antibodies in the body. Ginseng stimulates memory, counteracts fatigue, and soothes damage caused by stress. It may also increase stamina and well-being. Unlike other natural stimulants, ginseng usually does not cause irritability, addiction, or anxiety.

- Available in tea, powder, capsules, tablets, and extract.
- Side effects include headaches, insomnia, anxiety, breast soreness, or skin rash. More serious problems include asthma

attacks, heart palpations, increased blood pressure, or uterine bleeding. Do not take if you are pregnant. If you take an MAO for depression, avoid ginseng.

Gotu kola (*Centella asiatica*).   Improves mental ability. Some proponents of gotu kola claim that it eases the stress response.
- Available as leaves, capsules, or extract.
- Side effects may include skin rash or gastrointestinal complaints. Do not use if you are pregnant or nursing.

Ginkgo (*Ginkgo biloba*).   Protects cell membranes from free radical damage, improves concentration and memory, increases blood flow and helps the symptoms of PMS and depression. It is used to help with short-term memory loss and other problems of aging.
- Available in capsules, dried root, and prepared herbal tea.
- May cause nausea, diarrhea, stomach upset, and vomiting in larger doses and reduces clotting time. If you are taking coumadin, do not take this herb.

Herbal Mood Lifter

St. John's wort (*Hypericum perforatum*), the popular herbal remedy used to lift symptoms of depression, is taken by more than 20 million Germans on a daily basis and has become quite popular in the United States. This herbal supplement is taken internally to relieve depression without the side effects of prescription antidepressants.

In a study published in the *British Journal of Obstetrics and Gynaecology* (July 2000), researchers report that St. John's wort may help women with PMS (premenstrual syndrome) by easing nervous tension, anxiety, depression, and insomnia.

St. John's Wort is available as capsules, tincture, extract, oil, and dried leaves and flowers. St. John's Wort can cause sensitive skin in sunlight. Moreover, because this herb can interact with prescription medications, talk to your doctor before self-medicating. (Caution: Since the mechanism of action of St. John's wort is uncertain, using it with antidepressants such as monoamine oxidase inhibitors and selective serotonin reuptake inhibitors is not advised. Pregnant women are advised not to take St. John's wort.)

Calming Herbs

When any type of chronic pain robs you of sleep, you awaken feeling frazzled and anxious. The following herbs may sufficiently calm you down without causing you to feel "drugged."

Chamomile (*Matricaria recutita*).   Depresses the central nervous system and may also aid in boosting immune power. This healing herb is said to increase relaxation and promote quality sleep. It can be used to relieve nervousness, upset stomach, and menstrual cramps.
- Available as dried herb, supplements, and herbal tea.
- May cause problems for those allergic to ragweed, although there are no reports of toxicity.

Kava (*Piper methysticum*).   Relaxes muscles and has a sedative effect on the body. It is a member of the pepper family and has been used in the South Pacific as a natural relaxant. Kava has been reported to help long-term memory, muscle contractibility, insomnia, and anxiety, including the stresses of daily life. It is used as an anti-inflammatory or as a pain reliever to replace aspirin, acetaminophen, or ibuprofen.
- Available as tea or tincture, and in tablet form.
- Side effects may include muscle weakness, visual impairment, dizziness, and drying of the skin. Long-term use of the herb can contribute to hypertension, reduced protein levels, blood cell abnormalities, or liver damage. Alcohol consumption increases the toxicity of the herb. Do not use if pregnant, nursing, or being treated for depression or Parkinson's disease.

Passion flower (*Passiflora incarnata*).   Gives a mild tranquilizer effect and helps ease insomnia, stress, and anxiety.
- Available as tincture, fruit, dried or fresh leaves, or capsules.
- Avoid combining passionflower with prescription sedatives, and do not take if pregnant or nursing.

Valerian (*Valeriana officinalis*).   Has a sedative effect and has been shown to help in treating insomnia. It is also used to relieve high anxiety, stress, and nervousness.
- Available as capsules, tincture, and dried flowers.
- Avoid taking if you already take prescription antidepressants; may cause stomach upset.

Herbal Rubs and Tinctures

Some herbs work best to relieve pain when they are rubbed into the painful joints or muscles. Here are the most popular herbal salves. They can be found at health food stores and most drug stores.

Arnica (*Arnica montana*). The active components in arnica are *sesquiterpene lactones*, which are known to reduce inflammation and decrease pain. In ointment form, arnical tincture acts as an anti-inflammatory and analgesic for aches and bruises. Arnica may cause a skin rash in some people and should not be taken internally, as it can increase blood pressure and may damage the heart muscle.

Capsicum (*Capsicum frutesens*). The ointment made from the spice in cayenne pepper is an effective treatment for muscle spasms, tension headaches, osteoarthritis, rheumatoid arthritis, fibromyalgia, and back or neck pain. It is also used to relieve pain caused by shingles and surgical scars. Capsaicin, the active ingredient in capsicum, temporarily stimulates the release of substance P in the nerves. This may initially result in pain and burning, but repeated applications deplete substance P, which limits the ability of the nerves to transmit sensations and reduces pain. It's best to use disposable gloves to apply three to four times daily, and if you feel you need to get it off once it's been applied, wipe the area with a *dry* cloth. (If you wet the area, it may burn more.) Wash your hands well after use to avoid getting in your eyes, nose, mouth, or private parts.

Capsicum is available as *Capsaicin* and *Zostrix;* both are nonprescription drugs and are available at most pharmacies and grocery stores.

Dietary Supplements

A decade ago, the most popular dietary supplement was a vitamin/ mineral supplement. Herbal ingredients were scarce, and most people hadn't heard of tablets such as glucosamine, the popular arthritis pain reliever made from shrimp, crab, and lobster shells. Today in the United States, dietary supplements include a wide assortment of products, including multivitamins, minerals, amino acids, herbs, with ingredients derived from both plant and animal sources. These are available in an assortment of forms from capsules, pills, and gel tabs to liquids, tinctures, extracts, and powders.

While the dietary supplement industry is not regulated by the Food and Drug Administration (FDA), in 1994 the FDA established standards for manufacturers assuring that supplements bear ingredient and nutritional labeling. For instance, according to the FDA, herbal supplements must state the part of the plant from which the ingredient is derived. An herbal supplement such as black cohosh, commonly taken to decrease symptoms of menopause, might state on the label "Black Cohosh extract (root) containing 2.5 percent Triterpene Glycosides . . . 160 mg. (milligrams). Other ingredients: Rice Powder, Silicon Dioxide, Magnesium Stearate, Gelatin." Other than that, manufacturers are free to make whatever claims they want on the supplement label or in literature, and there is no assurance that these claims are valid. That's why you need to be cautious when choosing dietary supplements, including herbal remedies.

Glucosamine

The natural over-the-counter supplement glucosamine works for many women in alleviating the pain and stiffness of arthritis. In the body, glucosamine is a naturally occurring amino sugar found in human joints and connective tissues. The body uses it for cartilage development and repair. The supplement form of glucosamine comes from crab, lobster, and shrimp shells and has been found to help maintain lubrication in the joints, stimulate cartilage repair chemistry, and slow the breakdown of cartilage. In a host of studies, the outcome continues to be the same: glucosamine can relieve the symptoms of osteoarthritis at least as effectively as some commonly used NSAIDs.

Evidence published in the January 2001 issue of *The Lancet*, a British medical journal, confirmed that glucosamine may even slow the progression of osteoarthritis. In the study, 212 people with osteoarthritis were randomly selected to receive either 1500 milligrams of glucosamine each day or a placebo (sugar pill). Researchers concluded that those patients who took glucosamine experienced far less wear and tear of the joints than those who took the placebo. This is especially good news for people who are aspirin sensitive or who cannot take NSAIDs because of allergy or gastrointestinal upset.

Because glucosamine is an unregulated dietary supplement, the quality of the product will vary. Glucosamine is available in capsules, tablets, analgesic gel, and liquid form. Do not take if you are pregnant or allergic to shellfish.

Chondroitin Sulfate

Chondroitin sulfate is another popular over-the-counter supplement that many women use successfully to ease osteoarthritis symptoms. Some studies show that chondroitin reduces joint pain significantly and that overall mobility is significantly greater with this supplement. Like glucosamine, chondroitin sulfate appears to be safe and effective for treating arthritis symptoms. There are no studies, however, showing that both supplements are necessary for pain relief, even though manufacturers often mix the two supplements in over-the-counter pain formulas.

Chondroitin is available in capsules and tablets. There are no known side effects.

SAM-e

The preliminary study results behind SAM-e (S-adenosyl methionine) are quite promising, as this dietary supplement is thought to have anti-inflammatory, pain-relieving, and tissue-healing properties. At least one large study of SAM-e found similar benefit to naproxen, a common nonsteroid anti-inflammatory drug (NSAIDs) prescribed to relieve pain and inflammation. Yet, unlike naproxen or other NSAIDs, SAM-e has fewer side effects. During clinical trials of SAM-e as a treatment for depression, some patients reported marked improvement in their osteoarthritis.

Researchers also believe that SAM-e raises levels of the neurotransmitter dopamine, which is vital for mood regulation. While SAM-e is not as powerful as St. John's wort, according to research, the mood elevation and anti-inflammatory effects are felt in the body much faster, within a few days.

European doctors have prescribed SAM-e for more than twenty years for depression and pain. I recommend SAM-e to some patients who cannot tolerate NSAIDs. Many are able to maintain an active lifestyle using this natural supplement and can avoid the added expense (and side effects) of stronger medications. As with all dietary supplements, do not overuse SAM-e. Follow the package directions, and if you are taking other medication, talk to your doctor before using this supplement.

5-Hydroxytryptophan (5-HTP)

This over-the-counter supplement effectively increases the central nervous system (CNS) synthesis of serotonin. As discussed previously, serotonin levels have been implicated in depression, anxiety, pain sensation, and sleep regulation. In a study published in the October 1998 issue of *Alternative Medicine Review*, researchers reported that supplementation with 5-hydroxytryptophan (5-HTP) has been shown to improve symptoms of depression, anxiety, insomnia, and somatic pains in a variety of patients with fibromyalgia.

Essential Fatty Acids

Essential fatty acids are essential to the immune system because they seem reduce inflammation associated with allergic response by multiple mechanisms. Fish oils appear to diminish the generation of potent pro-inflammatory prostaglandins, resulting in anti-inflammatory effects. Essential fatty acids are available in oils containing omega-3 (fish oils) and omega-6 (linolenic and gamma-linolenic (GLA), which are found in plant oils such as evening primrose, black currant, and borage.

In the past, the omega-3 fatty acids in fish oil (eicosapentaenoic acid or EPA) were used primarily for relief of rheumatoid arthritis (RA) because RA involves significant inflammation and these fatty acids have anti-inflammatory effects. However, we now know that other types of chronic pain also have inflammation, so EPA may help to reduce this.

It is important to use EPA in addition to your basic treatment program, *not* to replace it. When used in doses recommended on the label, no serious side effects are known. These fatty acids enable the body to make more products that tend to decrease the inflammation. Eicosapentaenoic acid is available in capsules without a prescription at your drug store or health food store. It takes twelve to sixteen weeks of EPA therapy before benefits begin.

Vegetarians who want to gain this anti-inflammatory benefit can substitute borage seed oil, black currant oil, flaxseed or flaxseed oil, or evening primrose oil—all said to be helpful in offsetting the inflammation caused by arthritis. In a study conducted at Shriner's Hospital for Children in Boston, participants suffering with rheumatoid arthritis responded favorably to treatment with gamma-linolenic acid (GLA). This offers new hope for treating these serious inflammatory diseases with natural products, including foods.

Super Malic for Fibromyalgia and Arthritis

Malic acid, derived from the food you eat, may play a key role in energy production, especially for those with arthritis and related diseases. In several studies, patients with fibromyalgia (FMS) and other types of arthritis took malic acid. Within forty-eight hours of supplementation, almost all had improvement in pain. Likewise, upon discontinuation of malic acid for forty-eight hours, the improvement was lost.

Super Malic, a tablet containing malic acid (200 mg) and magnesium (50 mg), is being studied for treatment of fibromyalgia or deep muscle pain and overall aching. In scientific studies, volunteers with FMS took a fixed dose of Super Malic. While no symptom change was seen in short-term trials, when the dose was increased (up to six tablets of Super Malic, twice a day) and continued for a longer duration of treatment in the open label trial, some reductions in the severity of pain and tenderness were found. (An open label trial is one in which the medication is not blinded, meaning the drug is known to both the investigator and the participant.)

Researchers believe that Super Malic is safe and may be helpful in treating arthritis and fibromyalgia. If you try Super Malic with your doctor's consent, consider staying on this therapy for at least two months to receive the full benefit.

Bromelain

A natural protein-digesting enzyme found in pineapple (*Iananas comosus*), bromelain has an anti-inflammatory effect in the body that may help to ease many types of pain, including arthritis, fibromyalgia, TMJ, tension or sinus headaches, and carpal tunnel syndrome. In uncontrolled studies, bromelain supplements were found to give some relief to rheumatoid arthritis patients, including reduced pain and swelling. Because bromelain dissolves damaged scar tissue and speeds the healing rate of bruises, it is helpful for those who suffer frequently with tendonitis or sports related injuries such as tennis elbow. Bromelain works in the body by inhibiting the release of certain inflammation-causing chemicals. It is available in tablet or capsule form for supplementation use, and should be taken bucally (dissolved between your gum and the inside of your cheek).

Papain

Papaya contains papain, another proteolytic enzyme that is the key ingredient in meat tenderizer. Like bromelain, papain helps the body break down protein and is useful to decrease inflammation. Both bromelain and papaya supplements can be found at most drug or health food stores and should be taken bucally (dissolved between your gum and the inside of your cheek).

Bioflavonoids

The plant-derived bioflavonoids, often found in combination with vitamin C, have strong antioxidant and anti-inflammatory properties and appear to modulate key enzyme reactions in the inflammatory response. Bioflavonoids are found in green tea, citrus fruit, berries, onions, and stone fruits. Available supplemental bioflavonoids include rutin, quercetin, hesperidin, and proanthocyanidins (especially grape seed oil). All affect the structure of collagen, protecting it from free radical destruction and cross-linking directly with the collagen fibers.

Aromatherapy

I believe there is some benefit to using various aromas to help distract you from pain. These essences or oils have beneficial healing powers, helping reduce anxiety, combat stress, fight infection, increase productivity, or serve as a powerful aphrodisiac. There are studies showing that lavender increases the alpha wave activity in the back of the brain, which can help lead to relaxation and feelings of contentment. Increased beta activity in the front of the brain shows greater alertness and is said to occur with the scent of lemon.

If you use therapeutic massage with aromatherapy oils, you can heighten the healing effect. There are numerous aromas, oils, and essences that are used with touch or energy-based therapies to reduce stress, anxiety, and insomnia, as well as to support healing.

For example, some patients claim that rubbing a dilution of peppermint (*Mentha piperita*) oil on a painful muscle has a momentary numbing effect. For decades, people have used dilutions of wintergreen (*Gaultheria procumbens*) oil to ease aching muscles or lower back pain. Wintergreen oil may have an analgesic effect, as it contains methyl salicylate, an ingredient similar to that found in aspirin.

Essential Oils Are Highly Concentrated and Aromatic

Essential oils are highly concentrated substances (75 to 100 times more concentrated than the oils in dried herbs) extracted from a variety of different parts of a plant, including the flower, bark, roots, leaves, wood, resin, seeds, or rind (in the case of citrus fruits).

How to Use Essential Oils

- Inhale the oil by adding 5 to 10 drops to steaming water or to a humidifier.
- Mix 1 teaspoon with 1 pint carrier oil (sesame, borage, mineral, or olive) and use as a massage oil.
- Add 5 to 10 drops to warm bath water.
- Mix 5 drops with 1 cup warm water and mist into the air.
- Put 1 to 2 drops on top of a candle's melted wax, and inhale the warm scent.
- For ankle or foot pain, add 4 drops of lemon balm (*Melissa officinalis*) oil to a small tub of warm water and soak your lower legs and feet for twenty minutes.
- For PMS or anxiety, add 4 drops of lavender (*Lavendula officinalis*) oil to a warm bath and let the fragrance help relax your nerves.
- For migraine or tension headache or neck pain, put a few drops of peppermint *(Mentha piperata)* oil in a warm tub of bath water and soak for twenty minutes.
- Place a tissue scented with lavender oil under your pillow to help sleep easier.

Physical Medicine

Splints Let the Joint Rest

If your pain stems from an injury, your doctor may recommend a collar, splint, or brace for a short period to allow the injury to heal.

For instance, women with arthritis, bursitis, or carpal tunnel syndrome may find splints or supports helpful when pain flares. These splints are lightweight, usually plastic with Velcro straps to make them easy to put on and take off.

In the hand, a lightweight splint can give rest to the joints while still allowing use of the hand and thumb. A soft cervical collar for the neck may be helpful when back or neck pain flares. If the pain is severe or travels down one of the arms or leg, you should see your doctor to find the cause of the pain.

If you suffer from TMJ, headaches, or other facial pain, your doctor might use an occlusal (bite) splint to help reposition the temporomandibular joint. If properly done, the occlusal splint can alleviate facial and jaw tension, improve muscle balance, and boost blood flow in major areas of the body.

Proper Shoes Support the Body

Be sure your shoes are not adding to your pain. For pain in the feet or ankles, shoes can give extra support and make walking easier. Nevertheless, if shoes are too tight or if there are areas of excess pressure, then the feet can be an extra source of pain. Studies by the American Academy of Orthopaedic Surgeons show that 43 million Americans have foot problems. In a survey by the American Academy of Orthopaedic Surgeons, 80 percent of women said their feet hurt; almost 60 percent said they wore uncomfortable shoes at least an hour each day.

So, what kind of shoe is best? In a comprehensive study published in the April 2001 issue of *The Lancet*, researchers reported that high-heeled shoes with chunky heels are just as bad on your knees as stiletto heels, increasing pressure on the inside of the knee. I recommend that patients change to a sturdy flat shoe in order to decrease knee pain and be active again. Studies show that most women wear their shoes too small, which can greatly increase pressure on the feet and ankles, resulting in damage. To end pain, you need to wear shoes that support your weight yet don't put abnormal pressure on joints. When your weight distribution is improved, excess forces on the knees and hips are reduced and pain is improved.

Depending on your type of pain, your doctor may prescribe orthotics, specially designed inserts that are put inside your shoes, which help alleviate heel or ankle pain. Specialty shoe stores have these available, or the insert can be made specifically for your foot and problem.

Sleep Better ... Naturally

We know that chronic pain causes people to lose sleep. This loss of sleep can magnify the pain messages that are sent throughout your body. When the pain-sleep cycle happens frequently, it becomes vicious and is hard to break without some intervention. Not only is attention to sleep hygiene important, but also such stimulants as caffeine and nicotine must be avoided. Regular daily exercise, including stretching and aerobic activity, can help to consolidate sleep and to alleviate other pain symptoms.

High levels of arousal associated with racing thoughts, worrying or rumination may also delay sleep onset, or worries may cause you to have restless sleep or wake up early. Meditation or guided imagery (see Step 6) can help you relax at night as you learn to focus your thoughts on a neutral or enjoyable target. Some herbs and supplements that might help you relax include the following:

- Kava (*Piper methysticum*) helps end insomnia and anxiety, including the stresses of daily life. See page 168 for more on kava.
- Passion flower (*Passiflora incarnata*) has mild sedative properties and can help to alleviate insomnia. See page 168 for more on passion flower.
- Valerian (*Valeriana officinalis*) relieves insomnia or disrupted sleep habits by calming nerves and easing nervous tension. See page 168 for more on valerian.
- Melatonin (natural hormone) helps to cause a "phase shift" of the sleep cycle and may help raise levels of serotonin, which increases calmness.

Change Lifestyle Habits

You can alleviate some pain by making much-needed changes in the way you work and play. For instance, if you suffer with carpal tunnel syndrome, stretching or flexing your fingers and arms periodically while working at a computer can help alleviate the tension you feel. Also, modify the way you do daily activities to avoid putting pressure on your injured wrists. If you use a computer, make sure you have a proper wrist rest.

While you are changing your habits, be sure to watch the way you lift and carry heavy items. A study published in the December

2001 issue of the *Journal of Rheumatology* shows heavy lifting on the job can triple your risk of developing osteoarthritis in one or both of your hips. So when you lift an object from the floor, hold the object close to your body (lifting with the arms held out away from your body puts higher amounts of stress on the back). Also, lift with your legs and not your back. This uses the strength of the legs to help take the load off the back muscles. Avoid lifting objects higher than chest level as this can cause much higher stress on the back muscles.

Exercise

The benefits of exercise in helping you end pain are discussed in the next step of my program, as physical activity is a natural therapy for keeping you fit. Even adding a twenty- to thirty-minute walk, three times a week, can help alleviate your pain, increase the quality of your sleep, and boost your mood.

Stop Smoking

Another key lifestyle change that can decrease pain is stopping cigarettes. Not only is smoking a risk factor for most major diseases, such as cancer, cardiovascular disease, and diabetes, some research suggests that nicotine in the smoke might worsen some types of pain. For instance, smoking increases menstrual cramping by constricting blood vessels in your uterus. Smoking is also a risk factor in some types of headache, vascular problems, and for osteoporosis.

Will giving up smoking help to resolve your pain? The only way you'll know for sure is to give up smoking for several months. Moreover, by that time, even if you didn't get pain relief, I hope you'd consider giving up cigarettes altogether to preserve your health and longevity.

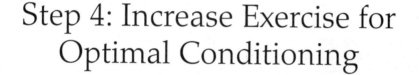

CHAPTER TWELVE

Step 4: Increase Exercise for Optimal Conditioning

When Denise was diagnosed with rheumatoid arthritis fifteen years ago, she was told to avoid physical activity because it might further damage her painful joints. Joan received the same recommendation from her family doctor when, at age seventeen, she sought treatment for painful menstrual cramps. "He told me to get in bed with a heating pad that time of the month and don't move around much because that could increase the cramping."

In the not too distant past, doctors did recommend complete bed rest for women who complained of migraines, back or neck pain, and other types of chronic pain. Until recently, many doctors felt that exercise might exacerbate symptoms of chronic pain, so they encouraged patients to refrain from too much activity. However, in the past decade, researchers have become increasingly aware of the importance of conditioning exercise and activity to increase fitness, strengthen bones and muscles, and ease most types of chronic pain conditions. While rest is important for most women with pain, especially during flare-ups, you must balance rest with daily physical activity in order to stay fit and increase overall health.

The Miracle Cure—and It's Free

When you engage in a comprehensive fitness program, consisting of cardiovascular (aerobic) exercise, stretching (flexibility), and resistance (strengthening) exercise, you will improve your fitness and most likely reduce your pain. Aside from the proven cardiovascular benefits of exercise, check out the following ways exercise may benefit women with chronic pain:

- Improved sleep quality
- Weight control
- Prevention of bone loss
- Increased energy level
- Countered anxiety and depression
- Increased muscle strength
- Relief for stress and tension
- Improved body posture
- Maintenance of range of motion in the joints
- Decrease tension

Exercising regularly can help women with chronic pain actually decrease pain as they unwind, de-stress, lose weight, increase range of motion (the normal amount your joints can be moved in certain directions), and build muscle and bone strength. For women who suffer with tension headaches, exercise can help to reduce muscle tension and boost endorphins, the body's natural pain relievers. Perhaps one of the immediate benefits of exercise is the psychological boost you get with a decrease in anxiety and tension, an improvement of mood and well-being, and a general state of relaxation.

DAILY RX

To help reduce chronic pain, integrate a mixture of daily exercises, including:

- Stretching
- Weight lifting or resistance training, including using machines, resistance bands, or even canned foods from the kitchen pantry
- Walking or other aerobic activity
- Enjoyable activities, such as gardening or riding a bicycle

Exercise Improves Physical Function

There is a growing body of evidence that links exercise with reduced pain and better management of painful conditions, such as arthritis, osteoporosis, fibromyalgia, and even menstrual cramps. Different types of exercise can improve range of motion, function, strength, and endurance, resulting in reduced pain. Take fibromyalgia, for example. While this arthritis-related syndrome has no cure, researchers have found that exercise can improve physical function in patients—and improve mood. In a study published in the April 2002 issue of *Arthritis Care and Research*, researchers found that a combination of strength training and aerobic exercise, improved women's muscle strength and overall endurance. In the twenty-week study, the women underwent a progressive exercise regimen, starting with pool exercises to improve joint movement. They also walked and did resistance exercises with hand weights, machines, and their body's own resistance. At the end of the program, fibromyalgia patients reported that their overall strength and endurance levels improved, as did their moods, outlook, and pain.

Weight-Bearing Exercise Wards Off Fractures

Another excellent example of the impact of exercise—and the detriment of its absence—is with osteoporosis. More than 80 percent of the 30 million Americans with osteoporosis are women. Unfortunately most women do not realize that the more exercise they get, particularly weight-bearing exercise such as walking, the stronger their bones will be and the less likely they are to get osteoporosis or painful fractures. In a study published in the June 2001 issue of the *American Journal of Epidemiology*, researchers concluded that moderate levels of physical activity could help to prevent hip fractures. And no matter how active you once were, if you become inactive, you are at a higher risk for painful fractures. If you want to prevent osteoporosis and incapacitating fractures, it's important to *stay active your entire life*.

If you have rheumatoid arthritis, keeping bones strong is important, as you have a twofold increased risk of osteoporosis and the painful fractures because of low bone mass. In a study published in the April 2002 issue of the *Annals of the Rheumatic Diseases*, researchers found that women with rheumatoid arthritis who had the thickest thigh muscles also had thighbones that were denser and stronger. This finding supports the importance of exercise for women with rheumatoid arthritis to keep muscles and bones strong and to prevent painful and debilitating fractures.

Exercise does not have to be excessive or strenuous to stop or reverse bone loss. Two studies involving more than 800 older adults found that those who walked the equivalent of at least twenty to thirty minutes per day had much denser bones than inactive adults. Numerous studies have all made similar conclusions—weight-bearing exercise, such as walking, can stimulate bone mass to stay strong in women of all ages. This type of activity puts vertical force on the bones. This force creates mini-electrical currents that help to strengthen the bone being stressed. Excellent forms of weight-bearing exercises are:

Aerobics	Racket sports
Biking	Rowing
Dancing	Running
Jogging	Strength training

Women with Arthritis Improve with Exercise

If you have arthritis, you will benefit greatly from exercise, particularly weightlifting. A study conducted at Tufts University found that people with rheumatoid arthritis could safely increase their strength by up to 60 percent with a modest training program. Another study, published in the *Journal of the American Medical Association*, also reported improvements in osteoarthritis when patients combined weight training with aerobic exercise.

Depending on your type of arthritis, the following exercises can help to keep your joints healthy:

Aerobics (low impact)	Stretching
Biking (takes pressure off knee and ankle joints)	Swimming
	Tai chi
Knitting (hands)	Walking
Playing piano (hands)	Yoga
Resistance training	

Exercise Boosts Mood and Decreases Fatigue

Along with increasing muscle strength and endurance and keeping your muscles and joints active and healthy, exercise helps women with chronic pain de-stress, which may ease pain and improve sleep. Regular participation in aerobic training has been reported to reduce symptoms of moderate depression and enhance psychological fitness. Exercise can even produce changes in certain chemical levels in the body, which can have an effect on the psychological state. Studies that have focused on "depressed mood," as opposed to the more serious clinical depression, have found that just one hour of aerobic exercise helps to boost mood and give exercisers a sense of achievement. In a study reported in the January 2001 issue of the *Journal of Sports Medicine and Physical Fitness*, the "depressed-mood" group noticed a significant reduction in anger, fatigue, and tension, along with a boost in vitality and vigor. This study confirms what many women with chronic pain have experienced: that exercise is necessary to help them cope with the emotions of pain, as well as to reduce fatigue that may accompany their pain-related ailment.

Scientists from the United Kingdom have targeted a brain chemical that may help explain the connection between exercise and increased mood. The researchers found that aerobic activity seems to boost the body's levels of phenylethylamine, a chemical that is linked to energy, mood, and attention. In the study, published in the September 2001 issue of the *British Journal of Sports Medicine*, twenty healthy young men ran on a treadmill for thirty minutes. After the participants completed the exercise, researchers reported the average concentration of phenylethylamine in the participants' urine increased 77 percent.

Phenylethylamine is similar in some ways to amphetamines and may play a key role in what is known as the "runner's high." A *National Health and Nutrition Examination Survey* found that physically active people were half as likely to be depressed a decade later as those who were inactive.

Exercise Boosts Serotonin

Other research suggests that exercise may boost serotonin levels in the brain, resulting in a calming, anxiety-reducing effect, and in some cases, drowsiness. A stable serotonin level in the brain is associated with a positive mood state or feeling good over a period of time. We know that women may have a greater sensitivity to changes in serotonin, which is often indicated by mood swings during the menstrual cycle. Female hormones also act on the neurotransmitter serotonin following the birth of a child or during menopause.

Inactivity and lack of exercise can aggravate low serotonin levels. Not only does exercise act as nature's tranquilizer, helping to boost serotonin in the brain, but studies have shown that exercise also triggers the release of epinephrine and norepinephrine, which are known to boost alertness.

THE CYCLE OF INACTIVITY

Some patients question how exercise can actually improve mobility and decrease pain. In fact, many are afraid to move around more for fear it will worsen or increase their chronic pain, especially when they experience uncomfortable aches and pains during brief activity.

The problem arises when women with chronic pain first start their exercise program and experience the normal muscle aches at minimal levels of exertion. Many women experience a "cycle of inactivity" that begins with chronic pain, inactivity, poor fitness or physical conditioning, and then moves to fatigue and even more pain on exertion. Being inactive will increase the inefficiency of your muscles, making simple tasks seem painful and almost impossible. Muscles actually deteriorate or atrophy if not used. This results in loss of ability to exercise and more inactivity—a vicious cycle.

I believe most chronic pain patients have a reduced quality of life, which can be directly related to the result of other symptoms that impede activity, such as fatigue or depression. However, exercise and increased mobility are important components of a pain management plan to reduce the frequency of painful flares, improve endurance for daily activities, improve cardiovascular fitness, and improve coping skills. In other words, the more conditioned or fit you become, the more you can handle increased activity and have a better quality of life.

The Active Way to End Pain

While your ability to perform exercise may differ from others around you, no matter what type of pain you have, exercise will generally help you build strength and endurance, improve sleep patterns, provide a sense of well-being, and reduce depression and fatigue. Let's look at the types of exercise that can help end pain and increase your overall health.

Stretching

Stretching exercises help to elongate your muscles and prevent injury. Stretching not only improves circulation to the muscles and joints, it also increases your range of motion so that movement is easier. If you suffer with fibromyalgia, stretching can help alleviate the deep muscle pain and stiffness. If you have arthritis, stretching helps your joints keep their full range of motion and allows you to stay flexible. If you have painful menstrual cramps or back or neck pain, stretching can help ease muscle tension and pain. Talk to your doctor or physical therapist and ask for a complete list of range-of-motion exercises to decrease pain, tailored to your particular problem.

More than anyone, sedentary people need the relief from muscle tension and stiffness that stretching provides. Stretching, when done the right way, feels good. Improper or excessive stretching, however, may actually increase the likelihood of injury. Stretching requires no special shoes or equipment, and it can be done just about anywhere.

Start by stretching one muscle at a time. Hold your stretch for at least twenty to thirty seconds, and refrain from overdoing the stretch—you don't want to add more damage to your aching muscles or joints! It's all right to begin by doing just one or two repetitions of each stretching exercise. If you have joint or muscle pain, stretch in the morning after applications of moist heat or a warm shower, and then again at night after applications of moist heat or a warm shower.

As you increase your level of exercise and fitness, it's important to *not give up*. Think of your commitment to a daily exercise program as one positive step you can take to end chronic pain, and it takes time. The more you see your exercise time as equally important to your life as eating healthy food or taking medications, it will become easier, more natural, and a total part of your multifaceted program to help you feel good again.   The following is a suggested stretching program to help you increase flexibility and coordination. Start slowly, doing just a few repetitions the first week. As you progress, add more repetitions. If you feel increased pain, stop the exercise. If your pain does not subside, call your doctor.

TALK TO YOUR DOCTOR

To gain the strengthening benefit without causing further pain or injury, appropriate technique is very important. Talk with your physi-

Suggested Stretching Program to Increase Range of Motion and Flexibility

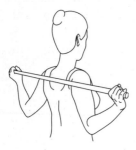

Chest and midback.   Place a broom handle or a long pole behind your back and across your shoulders with your hands supporting the long handle or pole at each end. Then slowly rotate your torso to the left; repeat this movement in the opposite direction.

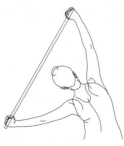

Shoulders.   Hold a broom handle or long pole over your head with both hands and slowly stretch from side to side like a pendulum several times. Then place the pole at shoulder level in front of you and gently turn to the right as far as it's comfortable, then to the left. Repeat several times.

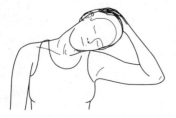

Neck.   Place one hand on the side of your head just above the ear and gently push as if you are trying to place your other ear to your shoulder. Gradually build pressure while allowing no movement of the head to occur. Hold and then relax.

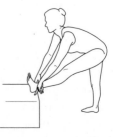

Legs and hamstrings.   Stand upright and put a foot on a bench or step. Slowly bend forward at the hip while keeping your back straight. Alternate to the other leg and repeat exercise. You should feel the stretch behind your thigh.

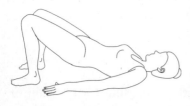

Back.   This exercise will help keep your posture straight and alleviate stress on the back and hips. Lie on your back with your knees bent and feet flat on the floor and hip-width apart. While contracting your abdominal muscles, press your lower back against the floor. You will feel your pelvis rock (tilt) toward your shoulders. The bottom of your buttocks and your pelvis will come slightly off the floor during the action.

cian, and consider consulting with a physical therapist so that you have a specific program planned with your special pain needs in mind.

Cardiovascular

Cardiovascular exercise uses repetitive motion and helps work your heart and build endurance. Cycling, walking, and swimming are all cardiovascular because they use large muscles and your heart rate increases with motion. Weight-bearing exercise, such as walking or jogging, also strengthens your bones because it forces them to bear weight.

The following are suggested cardiovascular exercises to help you boost overall health, burn calories and get lean, and increase positive mood. Start slowly, doing just five minutes at first unless you are already exercising regularly. As you progress, increase your endurance exercise time by one to two minutes each one to two weeks, until you are doing twenty to thirty minutes, three times a week. If you feel increased pain, stop the exercise. If your pain does not subside or recurs with each attempt at exercise, call your doctor.

SUGGESTED CARDIOVASCULAR EXERCISES

Aerobics (low or high-impact)
Badminton
Baseball
Basketball
Biking (both outdoors and indoors)
Dancing
Jogging
Walking (outdoor or indoor treadmill)

Mall walking
Rowing
Skating
Skiing
Swimming
Water aerobics
Volleyball

COUNT YOUR STEPS

If you find walking on a treadmill (or around your block) incredibly boring, try counting your steps. In a study published in the *American*

College of Sports Medicine Health and Fitness Journal, experts found that counting your steps as you walk can build confidence, increase fortitude, and improve the chance of success. They recommend using a pedometer, a small instrument that hooks onto your belt and measures your steps during exercise. When used during walking, you can see exactly how many steps you took. Researchers estimated that 2,000 steps equal 1 mile. If 2,000 steps are unreasonable, try to take 500 steps (one-quarter mile) or 250 steps (one-eighth mile) and then build from there. Some people listen to music, radio shows, or books on tape as they walk to diminish boredom.

TRY WATER EXERCISES

If you find that exercising on land increases joint or muscle pain, check out water aerobics and stretching programs at your "Y" or fitness center. Many women with fibromyalgia, arthritis, osteoporosis, and back or neck pain find water exercises help them stay fit and decrease pain. Because fibromyalgia is associated with soft tissue problems, water exercise reduces the amount of pressure on these areas. Make sure you exercise in a warm-water pool (about 83 to 88 degrees Fahrenheit), to help warm muscles and joints and decrease pain (unless you have multiple sclerosis).

Resistance

Resistance exercise targets certain muscle groups and helps increase endurance and strength. Many women still associate weight training with building bulky muscles, but this is simply not true. Weight training will strengthen and preserve the muscle mass you already have and reduce the aches you feel with chronic pain ailments such as fibromyalgia, arthritis, back and neck pain, and more.

Your muscles are made up of bundles of fibers. You generally do not increase the number of fibers, but by exercising the muscles you can strengthen them. Resistance training forces an increase in muscle mass by subjecting it to a load it's not used to handling.

If you want to lose weight during exercise, resistance exercise will speed up the process. Muscle mass is metabolically active tissue (it burns calories), and the more muscle mass your body has, the more calories you burn all day, even while you are watching TV or chatting with friends on the Internet. Fat burns two to three calories per pound while muscle burns fifty calories per pound—and strength training will help you turn weak muscles into healthy, strong ones.

RELIEVE JOINT PAIN   A revealing study conducted at Tufts University found that people with rheumatoid arthritis could safely increase their strength by up to 60 percent with a modest training program. Another study, published in the *Journal of the American Medical Association*, also found improvements in arthritis when patients combined weight training with aerobic exercise. To gain the strengthening benefit without irritating the joints, proper technique is important so as not to cause further injury. Check with your physician or consult with a physical therapist to help design an exercise program that meets your specific arthritis needs.

IT'S NEVER TOO LATE   If you think you're too old to lift weights, the latest findings conclude that this is not true. In a revealing study published in the January 2002 issue of *Medicine and Science in Sports and Exercise*, researchers studied sixty healthy men and women between the ages of sixty and eighty-three who engaged in either high-intensity resistance training using machines or low-intensity resistance training. In addition, a control group participated that did not change their lifestyle habits. After six months, the high-intensity group made significant improvement in bone density measurements where the thighbone meets the hip. This is the area (the femoral neck) where serious or even deadly fractures occur in older adults. Researchers believed that leg presses, overhead presses, and certain back-strengthening exercises had the most impact on boosting bone density.

The following is a suggested strength training or resistance program to help you build muscle strength and improve your posture. Concentrate on higher repetitions with less weight, which emphasizes tone and endurance rather than bulk. Resistance training also increases metabolism and boosts bone density.

Start slowly, doing just a few repetitions the first week. As you progress, add more repetitions gradually—one to two per week. If you feel increased pain, stop the exercise. If your pain does not subside, or recurs each time you attempt to exercise, call your doctor.

SUGGESTED RESISTANCE PROGRAM   You can use isometric exercises with resistance bands (found at most sporting goods stores) or free weights. These light, handheld weights are available at sporting goods stores. If you don't have free weights, use canned vegetables or beans. You can get the same resistance impact holding cans as you can with light weights. You can also buy light weights that can be strapped to your hand, wrist or ankle.

The American College of Sports Medicine advises a routine of eight to ten exercises, each with eight to twelve repetitions, at least twice a week. If you are a moderate exerciser, this minimal weight-training regimen will reap tremendous benefits for you. Use five-pound weights to start, and gradually increase this amount. Allow for ten minutes, three times a week, for resistance training. As you can accomplish the minimal regimen, gradually increase the following variables:

- Amount of weight
- Number of sets (a set is eight to twelve repetitions)
- Number of different exercises
- Amount of time spent exercising

EXAMPLES OF EXERCISES USING LIGHT WEIGHTS   Sitting in a chair, with a weight strapped at your ankle, straighten your knee out and lower it back down to the floor. Be sure to go only as far as is comfortable, and use only one-pound weights for this resistance exercise. Repeat once, then twice, and then gradually increase up to five or ten times twice daily, if you can do so without pain.

With the weight strapped around your wrist, raise your arm upward toward your head and then back to the side of your body. Repeat once, then twice, then gradually increase up to ten times, twice daily.

Arm circles can be done with a one-pound weight strapped around the wrist. Or, you can use handheld weights or even canned vegetables to get the same resistance. Start with a small circle, and then gradually increase the size of the circle. Repeat once, then twice, then gradually increase up to ten times twice each day, if possible.

Lying on your bed, slide one leg out to the side and back to the middle with the weight strapped just above the ankle. Do this for both legs. Repeat once, then twice, then gradually increase up to ten times twice each day as long as you can comfortably do to the repetitions without any pain.

PROTECT YOUR BACK WITH ABDOMINAL CRUNCHES

Strong abdominal muscles help keep your back strong and can ease chronic pain. To build strong abs, lie on your back with knees bent. Cross your arms across the chest and lift shoulders up so the shoulder blades clear the floor. Do five reps to start. Increase as you can without additional pain.

Daily Living Activities

If your life is too busy to stop and exercise each day, make sure you are moving around with household chores and daily living activities. I treated forty-two-year-old Kate, a childcare director and mother of four, for chronic tension headaches. Time was at a premium for Kate, so I suggested that she exercise by intentionally stretching while doing her household chores, and increase her walking time while shopping and playing with her children. Kate did just that, and also found gardening was an outdoor activity that she could enjoy with her children and benefit from the lifting, digging, pulling, bending, and other movements needed to cultivate the soil. She realized that the more she did in her garden, the less stress she felt and her tension headaches began to subside.

As you check the following list of beneficial activities, choose those that are pleasurable and that you will stick with—just make certain your body is in motion so you get a full workout. Depending on your personal fitness level, vary the exercises to keep from getting bored.

Active play with children
   or grandchildren
Climbing the stairs instead
   of using the elevator
Gardening
Housecleaning
Jumping rope
Mowing the lawn

Playing Frisbee
Playing softball or kickball
   with the family
Riding bikes with children
Vacuuming
Walking the dog
Window washing

Ancient Disciplines to Ease Pain and De-stress

Tai Chi

Tai chi, an ancient martial art used in China for more than 1,000 years, may give an added benefit to women who live with arthritis and deep muscular pain or any type of tension-related pain. In past clinical studies, experts concluded that tai chi helped ease arthritis symptoms and helped to build strength, balance and flexibility through gentle movements. Now findings published in the May 2001 issue of the journal *Annals of Behavioral Medicine*, concluded that tai chi could make healthy older adults better able to undertake an assortment of activities, such as walking, climbing stairs, and carrying groceries.

This ancient discipline with its deep-breathing component, is sometimes described as "moving meditation," as you relax using the various movements. Some studies have shown that adults who regularly do tai chi experienced greater spinal flexibility than those who do not. In addition, in one small study of older adults, ages sixty-eight to eighty-seven, those who regularly practiced tai chi reported less overall pain than those who did not do tai chi.

With tai chi, you follow a series of slow, graceful movements that mimic the movements you do in daily life. You move forward, backward, and from side to side in a carefully coordinated manner—flowing together as if your body is doing one continuous movement. Tai chi is said to speed healing, improve circulation, boost immune function, and decrease stress.

In findings reported at the American College of Rheumatology, in December 2001, researchers found that women with arthritis who did tai chi reported less pain, more comfort while doing daily activities, improved balance, and greater abdominal muscle strength. If you have arthritis, fibromyalgia, osteoporosis, or other back or neck pain, tai chi may help you manage pain and improve your balance so your daily activities are easier to accomplish. In addition, because of the focus on slow, flowing movement forward and backward, tai chi can help you increase balance without adding to pain in your muscles and joints.

You can purchase books and videos on tai chi and use them in the privacy of your home. On the other hand, you may enjoy the company of doing this with others at a local health spa or "Y".

Yoga

Yoga not only provides the benefit of relaxing your body, but its various positions can help improve your balance, flexibility, and overall health. Because chronic pain is influenced by emotions, thoughts, and behaviors, yoga's mind/body focus can be successfully used to ease pain and improve mental outlook. Through controlled breathing, prescribed postures (called *asanas*), and meditation, this ancient Indian practice allows you to experience *prana* (life force) from the inside out and achieve a true state of balance between body, mind, and spirit. Asanas exercise every muscle in the body.

Some of my patients enjoy yoga for exercise and stretching; others use it for stress reduction and meditation. Relaxation, flexibility, and muscle strength are all important outcomes of yoga, making it a good exercise for those who are unable to do more aerobic-type exercises. With yoga, there is no high impact or bouncing.

POPULAR SYSTEMS OF YOGA   *Bikram* yoga uses a precise system of postures to warm and stretch the body. When you attend a bikram yoga class, you will practice the same twenty-six postures in each class. You might find the room to be extremely warm, to help heat the muscles for deeper stretching. People often sweat profusely with bikram yoga.

With *vinyasa* or *astanga* yoga, you will "flow" from one posture to another in a series. Vinyasa helps to heat the body quickly, enabling the muscles to warm up. Practitioners of this style often develop strength rapidly, as the flow series can sometimes be demanding.

Another popular yoga system, *viniyoga*, incorporates coordinating the breath with the postures. With viniyoga, there is a strong focus on relaxation and moving with the breath. Many women find this style of yoga to be more nurturing and relaxing than others.

Of all the various systems, however, *iyengar* yoga may be the best for helping alleviate chronic pain. Findings from Harbor-UCLA Medical Center in Torrance, California, showed that iyengar yoga, which combines breathing exercises with difficult poses, may help even older adults alleviate chronic arthritis pain. With this system of yoga, you focus on exact alignment and precision in the yoga postures. The postures are held longer than in other yoga systems, as the breath-work encourages deeper stretching. If you are a beginner, you will start with standing postures. By learning how to stand, walk, and sit using the muscles correctly, you can improve your well-being and muscular tension. In some classes, you might use props, such as straps, blocks, or chairs, to help you relax or free areas that are extremely sore and tight. If you choose to study iyengar yoga, it helps to find a teacher who is certified.

No matter which system you study, the yoga postures should never intensify pain. If your pain worsens, stop immediately. A qualified instructor should work with you—and your type of pain—to help you find relief over time. The teacher should be well versed in anatomy and physiology, and have experience working with different health conditions.

TRY THE COBRA

To alleviate back or hip pain, try the cobra position: Lie face down on the floor, and place your palms against the floor under your shoulders. Gently push your chest up and away from the floor as you slowly inhale. Allow your shoulder blades to pull back together and your chest to extend forward and upward. Don't straighten your arms all the way when you first do this, especially if your hips lift off the floor. Hold this position for a few seconds, then, as you exhale, return to the starting position. Repeat three or four more times to gradually build strength.

Pilates

Pilates is another alternative form of exercise that has become increasingly popular, particularly among dancers. With pilates, you do a series of movements on special equipment under the supervision of a professional instructor. This method focuses on flexibility and works to "lengthen" your spine by lifting your rib cage and strengthening your abdomen. The improved posture will result in less pressure on painful joints.

Making Exercise Part of Your Life

How Much Is Enough?

While national guidelines recommend thirty minutes of physical activity daily as a minimum exercise requirement, researchers found in a study published in October 2001 in the *Journal of the American College of Nutrition* that exercising in three ten-minute bouts is equally effective in keeping you fit. Many patients find that it's easy to fit short exercise periods into their day and alternate between the various types of exercise, along with household chores and daily living activities.

Keeping a regular exercise journal is important as you start exercising for optimal conditioning and fitness. Purchase a calendar, and record the amount and type of exercise and activity performed each day, as well as the physical response, such as increased pain. This data can help you and your doctor design a specialized program that has optimum benefit without causing further pain or injury.

Be Comfortable

Exercise shoes are now sport specific, and it might take some time to find the right fit at the right price. Be sure to try on your shoes with the type of socks that you will be wearing to exercise, and make sure your toes have plenty of room in the toe box. Walk around in the store for a few minutes to see if the shoes rub or are uncomfortable in any way. If they are pinching now, just think how they will feel in the midst of your daily walk or bike ride.

Exercise as Social Support

Many times exercise classes or even walking the neighborhood with a special group of friends instead of exercising alone helps you stay with your program. The social support of friends or classmates encouraging you as you get through the daily routine can help your compliance with the program, as well as make it more fun.

Check with your local "Y" or fitness center for group exercise classes. Depending on the type of pain and your personal preference, you may find classes in low-impact aerobics, stretching, step aerobics, jazzercise, and more.

CHAPTER THIRTEEN

Step 5: Choose Healing Nutrients to Ease Your Pain

Food scientists continue to astound me with new discoveries on the therapeutic benefits of food. Not only do researchers theorize that certain foods may help decrease pain, they now claim that some nutrients in foods can reduce diseases that lead to pain. Take, for example, a study published in the March 2002 issue of *Arthritis and Rheumatism*. In this study, French scientists found that vitamin E can reduce joint destruction in mice with a specific rheumatoid-arthritislike condition. In another landmark study presented at the 2002 annual meeting of the American Pain Society in Baltimore, Maryland, researchers concluded that rats on a soy-based diet had less swelling and were able to tolerate more pain than another test group given a milk protein. As a doctor, I realize that we need more research to see if these outcomes work in humans. Nonetheless, the preliminary results are exciting and very promising for those who live with chronic pain.

Understanding the Food-Pain Connection

In chapter 1, I explained how scientists believe serotonin, the mood-elevating neurotransmitter, may reduce pain, decrease appetite, produce a sense of calm and relaxation, and induce sleepiness. Some researchers hypothesize that serotonin is involved in the regulation of carbohydrate intake. The theory suggests that too few carbohydrates result in reduced levels of serotonin, which can result in increased anxiety with disturbed sleep and a lower tolerance for pain. There are foods high in carbohydrates, such as breads, pasta, cereal, or sherbet, that might raise the level of serotonin in the brain.

Even though studies continue to point to a food-brain connection, finding the exact foods that help increase a feeling of calmness, decrease pain, and boost sound sleep relies on trial-and-error. No matter what type of pain you have, choose from the following list of high-carbohydrate foods to see which ones may give you pain relief and a feeling of calm.

FOODS TO BOOST SEROTONIN

Bagels	Muffins
Bananas	Pasta (plain)
Bread	Potatoes
Cereal	Rice
Crackers	Sherbet

Check Your Protein to Stay Alert

If pain leaves you feeling fatigued and lifeless, you may want to increase the amount of protein you eat, particularly foods like tuna, chicken, or turkey that are rich in an amino acid called tyrosine. When we eat protein food, this increases tyrosine, which boosts the levels of dopamine and norepinephrine, two brain neurotransmitters that increase a feeling of alertness and boost concentration.

Protein is also important in repairing body tissue and in fighting infection. Too little protein can lead to symptoms of weakness, apathy, and poor immunity. (The average-size woman needs about 45 to 55 grams of protein each day, but you may need more protein if you have fever or infection.)

One ounce of meat, chicken, cheese, or fish provides 7 grams of protein; 1 cup of milk, 8 grams of protein. Vegetable proteins, such as black beans or tofu, can make a good substitute for animal protein.

Make sure you include a protein source several times daily, particularly at times when you feel fatigued and need to clear your mind.

HIGH-PROTEIN FOODS RICH IN TYROSINE

Legumes and peas	Poultry
Beef	Soy products (soybeans,
Cheese	soy granules, soy milk, tofu)
Fish	Yogurt
Milk	

Avoiding Food Triggers

Fascinating personal testimony regarding food triggers and pain continues to surface each day. During patient consultations, women tell me of foods they avoid to decrease pain—and how this elimination method works for them. One patient, Kelly, found that avoiding yeast products helped ease the deep muscle pain of fibromyalgia. After staying off these foods for several weeks, Kelly said that when she ate pizza or cheese, she had muscle soreness the next day.

Kelly's food-pain discovery may have some validity, according to a report given in October 2001 at the American College of Nutrition in Orlando, Florida. In the study, researchers speculated that people with fibromyalgia might experience reductions in their symptoms simply by eliminating one or more foods from their diets. Fibromyalgia patients eliminated from their diet commonly eaten foods such as corn, wheat, dairy, citrus, soy, and nuts. After abstaining from these foods for two weeks, nearly half of the patients reported a significant reduction of pain. More than 75 percent had a reduction of symptoms such as headache, bloating, fatigue, and breathing difficulties. Patients then reintroduced certain foods every two or three days, and many had reactions such as pain or headache.

No matter what type of pain-related problem you have, the key to effectively managing the pain lies with your ability to recognize the triggers that provoke it. Once you identify the food triggers, remove them from your life. For instance, food scientists have identified chocolate, some types of cheese and dairy products, monosodium glutamate (MSG), nuts, citrus foods, meats, and alcohol (usually red wine) as possibly triggering migraine headaches. If you suffer with migraine headaches, I'm sure you're aware of this strong link between the food you eat and the onset or intensity of the migraine. Although the exact connection is unclear, it's thought that chemical sensitivities could lead to reactions in blood vessels and nerves that may increase the diameter of the blood vessels in the brain. These actions result in the pounding headache and other symptoms you feel. Some people with arthritis find eliminating foods in the nightshade family helps relieve symptoms. These foods include peppers, eggplant, tomatoes, and white potatoes. Other researchers believe that red meat, fruit, dairy products, and/or preservatives may increase pain in fibromyalgia and arthritis patients, if they are susceptible. Different studies have identified wheat and other grains in the diet as increasing arthritis pain. We know that salty foods and caffeine may increase PMS symptoms, including pain and bloating, in some women.

Try Food Elimination

So, how do you tell if a certain food triggers pain? While there are exact tests doctors can do, there is increasing proof that an elimination diet is most helpful in isolating and identifying pain triggers. With this diet, you eliminate the most common foods (see the following list) that may trigger a pain reaction for two weeks. When your pain symptoms subside, you slowly reintroduce these foods, one at a time, to see which ones might trigger symptoms.

Some of the most common foods you will eliminate at first may include:

Milk (butter, ice cream, yogurt, cheese, and other byproducts)

Wheat (all breads, crackers, cookies, noodles, and other by-products)

Corn (grits, popcorn, corn chips, corn syrups, corn starches, and by-products)

Citrus (oranges, grapefruits, lemons, limes, and other citrus and juices)

Berries (strawberries, blueberries, raspberries)

Eggs

Fish (shellfish, whitefish)

Peanuts (peanut butter or other products)

Tomato (pizza, spaghetti sauce, catsup, and tomato by-products)

Yeast (dried fruits, vinegar, mushrooms, bread, pickles, and others)

Soybeans (soy sauce, soy lecithin, tofu, and other soy products)
Carob
Chocolate
Colas, coffee, tea
Beans
Peas

The elimination diet usually allows the following foods:
Fresh poultry
Fresh meats
Vegetables (except the listed varieties)
Fruits (except the listed varieties)
Rice cereals
Water

After the two-week period, reintroduce the foods, one at a time. For example, if you are reintroducing corn, eat only a small amount of corn at first. If you have no reaction with the introduced food, then you can eat this food again in slightly larger amounts. You should also try byproducts of the food to see if these are well-tolerated. For instance, if you think corn products may trigger pain, be sure you test cornstarch, tortillas, or another byproduct. If there is no change in symptoms and you can tolerate the food, reintroduce another food. If you feel more pain, stop the new food immediately until the symptoms clear.

Use the food elimination diet under the careful supervision of a physician or licensed nutritionist to make sure you get adequate nutrition.

WATCH OUT FOR ADDITIVES

There is some evidence that fibromyalgia patients may feel less pain if they eliminate monosodium glutamate (MSG) and aspartame, which are found in many processed foods. Both additives may also be associated with migraine headaches and other chronic pain ailments. You should be aware of some processed foods that contain these ingredients, even though they may be listed under other names:

Autolyzed yeast

Calcium caseinate

Gelatin

Glutamate

Glutamic acid

Hydrolyzed protein

Monopotassium glutamate

Monosodium glutamate

Sodium caseinate

Textured protein

Yeast extract

Yeast food

Yeast nutrient

Maintaining a Normal Weight

Maintaining a normal weight is recommended for preventing or managing almost all types of chronic pain, especially to reduce back, hip, or knee pain, or the debilitating joint pain of arthritis. Being at a normal weight can also help those suffering with gynecological pain. Overweight women may have disruptions in their menstrual cycles due to an excess of androgens. There is also a correlation between being obese—20 percent or more over normal body weight—and the production of insulin, which can occupy the hormone receptor sites necessary for ovulation. Staying at a normal weight can help balance hormones and ease the pain of gynecological problems.

There is no doubt that living with chronic pain is stressful. Not only does it interrupt your sleep and force you to change your daily routine during painful flares, it can also take a toll on your waistline. My patients have said higher levels of pain leads them to crave comfort food that is salty, sugary, or greasy—like pizza, fudge brownies, or French fries. Especially when pain interferes with your relationships, causes you to miss social events, and literally robs you of quality of life, turning to comfort foods is normal reaction—but it's not going to ease your pain, and it may worsen it! In many cases, the heavier you are, the more pain you may feel. This is particularly true for joint and muscle pain.

How Much Should You Weigh?

Just how much should you weigh? Your weight can depend on many variables, including height, age, bone structure, and weight-cycling history. The best weight for you is the one that is closest to the recommended "normal" level and at which you can manage your chronic pain. Traditionally, height/weight charts gave an accurate portrayal of overweight. However, experts now believe that your body mass index (BMI) may give a more accurate picture of health. BMI is your body weight (in kilograms) divided by your height in meters squared. The BMI number or value correlates to your risk of adverse effects on health, with higher numbers showing an increased risk. According to the American Dietetic Association, people with a higher percentage of body fat tend to have a higher BMI than those who have a greater percentage of muscle.

Here's how to figure out your BMI:

1. Write down your weight in pounds _____.
2. Multiply that number by 703 (_____ × 703 = _____).
3. Multiply your height in inches by itself (_____ × _____ = _____).
4. Divide the answer to number 2 by the answer to number 3 to get your BMI _____.

BMI Categories

20–25	normal weight
26–29	overweight
30 and above	obese

Seven Simple Solutions to Lose Weight

Dieting is stressful, even without the added stress of living with constant pain. However, there are simple solutions that help my patients lose weight without too much effort. I believe your weight loss should occur over a period of months, losing no more than one to two pounds per week to make sure it stays off. Once they drop the first ten pounds, most of my patients notice a dramatic difference in the way they feel, with more energy, increased mobility, positive feelings, and improved productivity at home and at work. The more active you can be, the better you will sleep at night, and sound sleep helps ease pain. Try the following weight loss solutions that work for my patients:

1. *Stop dieting.*   Scientific studies have shed light on the impact of deprivation diets on weight loss, and the findings have consis-

tently held true: *Diets alone don't work.* In fact, if anything, dieting only makes you gain weight by training your body to store fat rather than burn it. While deprivation dieting can help you lose weight, for most women who eat less, one-third of this loss is reduction of muscle, not fat, and lean muscle (as opposed to body fat) is what helps burn calories. Studies show that fat burns two to three calories per pound while muscle burns fifty calories per pound. Muscle mass is metabolically active tissue, meaning that it is the tissue that burns calories. The more muscle mass your body has, the more calories you burn all day, even while you are sitting around.

2. *Focus on whole foods.* To lose weight or maintain a normal weight, I recommend eating plenty of low-fat, nutrient-dense foods such as fresh fruits and vegetables, beans, lentils, seeds, nuts, whole grain products, soy products, low-fat dairy, and fish. Let the foundation of your daily menu be on plant foods: fruits, vegetables, and grain products. You can use low-fat versions of some of these foods to complement the rest of the plant-based diet. Use fats and sweets sparingly, as they contribute extra calories but few nutrients.

3. *Use the glycemic index.* If you find yourself constantly hungry while trying to lose weight, try focusing on foods that are low on the glycemic index (GI). This is a numerical system that ranks carbohydrates on a scale of 0 to 100, according to their effect on blood glucose (sugar) levels. A food low on the glycemic index will cause a small rise in blood sugar; a food high on the glycemic index will trigger a more dramatic rise, which can cause an increase in appetite.

LOW GLYCEMIC INDEX FOODS

Low-fat dairy

Low-fat protein, tofu, nuts, legumes

Nonstarchy vegetables

Breakfast cereals based on wheat bran, barley, oats

Whole grain breads made with whole seeds

Barley, pasta, and rice instead of potatoes

Vinegar and lemon juice dressings

HIGH GLYCEMIC INDEX FOODS

Potatoes

Refined grains

Sweets

Vegetables high in starch (corn)

Candy

Pastries

---

4. *Watch your portion sizes.*   Portion sizes can make or break a weight reduction program, and unfortunately they seem to be increasing each year. For instance, the United States Department of Agriculture's recommended serving size for a cookie is half an ounce. Yet, the average cookie sold in restaurants is about 700 percent larger. Moreover, according to a study published in the February 2002 issue of the *American Journal of Public Health*, researchers found that portion sizes rose dramatically since the 1970s, and skyrocketed in the 1980s. They estimated that French fries, hamburgers, and cola drinks are now two to five times larger than their original sizes. Check the sidebar on pages 205–206 for accurate portion sizes, and then stay within this range to meet your normal weight goal.

5. *Limit the fat in your diet.*   While researchers used to believe that counting fat grams would allow you to lose weight, we now know this is *not* always the case. It is true that fat is calorie-dense and provides nine calories per gram. So, limiting foods loaded with fat automatically limits your calorie intake, leading to weight loss. Carbohydrate and protein, on the other hand, provide less than half the calories of fat or about four calories per gram. Nonetheless, eating as much as you want of low-fat or fat-free foods is not the answer to weight loss. If you eat more calories than you burn off, you still will gain weight.

   As you reduce fat in your diet, simply seek balance. Each individual food does not have to be 20 to 30 percent fat calories or less. Remember, fruits and vegetables have little or no fat while some foods, like low-fat cheese, may have 50 percent fat calories. The idea is to balance high- and low-fat foods over the course of the day and week.

While you are watching the fat content of your diet, recognize that the most important fats to stay away from are saturated fats and trans fatty acids. A diet high in saturated fat (the type of fat in meat and dairy products) and trans fatty acids (the type of fat in margarine, snack and fast-food products, crackers, pastries, and many processed foods) can lead to many types of cancer, obesity, and heart disease.

6. *Eat frequently.*   When most of my patients decide to lose weight, they tell me they simply stop eating. That lasts about one week until they are so ravenously hungry that they binge on anything in sight—and undo all their weight loss efforts. The best way to maintain a normal weight is to stop dieting and to eat more frequently—with nutritious minimeals. Dieting can often be hazardous to your health, as it restricts calories and nutritious foods, causing you to feel depressed and deprived, resulting in rebound binging or overeating. Contrary to deprivation dieting, eating *more frequently* will boost your metabolism and productivity. Research has found that people who eat two meals or less during the day have a slower metabolic rate (the speed at which your body burns calories, and the rate that we all want to go faster) versus those who eat three or more times a day. Eating frequently will also keep your blood glucose constant so that you do not feel irritable or overly hungry. Keeping blood sugar levels from having dramatic dips and rises can also help some women who suffer with PMS or migraine headache. Also, remember to drink plenty of water.

7. *Move around more.*   The best way to maintain or reach an ideal weight is to burn more calories than you take in through exercise and activity. Of dieters who are most successful at keeping off the weight, more than 95 percent are exercisers—and most are walkers. So, while you are busily figuring out your weight loss menu, make sure you include periods throughout the day when you get up and walk—whether around your yard, your apartment complex, your neighborhood, or the stairs at your office.

SAMPLE PORTION SIZES

Bread, Cereal, Rice, and Pasta

1 slice bread
½ hamburger bun (1 bun would equal two bread servings)

$\frac{1}{2}$ bagel (1 whole bagel would equal two bread servings)
$\frac{1}{2}$ English muffin
$\frac{3}{4}$ ounce pretzels
$\frac{1}{2}$ cup cooked cereal, pasta, or rice
1 ounce cold cereal

Fruit

1 medium piece of fruit
$\frac{1}{2}$ cup chopped, cooked, or canned fruit
$\frac{1}{2}$ cup fruit juice

Vegetables

$\frac{1}{2}$ cup cooked vegetables
1 cup raw vegetables

Milk

1 cup nonfat milk
1 cup nonfat, sugar-free yogurt
$1\frac{1}{2}$ ounce fat-free cheese

Meat and Meat Substitutes

2–3 ounces of lean meat, fish, or poultry without skin
1 to $1\frac{1}{2}$ cup cooked beans
2 eggs or $\frac{1}{2}$ cup low-cholesterol egg alternative

Ending Pain with Key Nutrients

We know there is a direct link between the food we eat and how we feel. So it makes sense that if you experience optimal health, eat a highly nutritious diet, and are able to exercise and be active, you may not feel pain as much as a woman who is sickly, inactive, and eats a poor diet. Furthermore, there is a lot we don't know about the micronutrients and other compounds in the foods we eat and their effects on the body. That is why you should focus on eating whole foods instead of popping megadoses of vitamins to help eliminate pain and stay well. I believe that every nutrient, micronutrient, and unknown compound in the food is equally important, and whole foods provide optimal healing nutrition.

Antioxidants and Phytochemicals Boost Disease Resistance

Eating a well-balanced diet of fresh fruits and vegetables high in antioxidants and phytochemicals can help maintain immune function and keep you well. An antioxidant is a super nutrient that helps repair cell damage and is vital to the body's resistance to infection. Phytochemicals are biologically active substances that give plants their color, flavor, odor, and protection against plant disease. Some phytochemicals work as potent antioxidants.

A Living Food Diet Has Helped Some

In a study published in the November 2000 issue of the journal *Toxicology*, researchers sought to see if a living food diet could help ease the swelling and pain of rheumatoid arthritis. Living food is an uncooked vegan diet, consisting of fruits, vegetables and roots, berries, nuts, germinated seeds, and sprouts. It is filled with the richest sources of vitamins C and E, and carotenoids. After eating the diet, patients showed higher levels of beta-carotene, lycopene and lutein, vitamins C and E, and polyphenolic compounds, such as quercetin, which has been shown to have an anti-inflammatory effect in the body. They also reported less pain and swelling, and increased mobility. When fibromyalgia patients went on the living food diet, they reported decreased joint stiffness and pain, as well as an improvement of their self-experienced health.

About Vitamins and Minerals

While all vitamins and minerals play a role in keeping us well, researchers have targeted specific nutrients which may influence pain. In this section I've highlighted those vitamins and minerals that could conceivably contribute to easing pain. While there are no guarantees these will work for every woman, I do know that good nutrition can help increase your energy and boost your immune system. If you are wondering, after reading the list, whether vitamin supplementation is necessary, check the following list. If you are in one or more of the categories, you may need to add a multi-vitamin/mineral supplement to your daily routine for some "nutrition insurance."

Women who are very busy and do not have time to eat properly.

Women who are allergic to dairy products or who do not drink milk.

Women of childbearing age who do not get ample folate in their diets.

Women who are on a very low calorie diet.

Women over age sixty-five who do not eat a balanced diet.

Women who are vegans and vegetarians.

Women who take daily medication.

Women with chronic illnesses.

Otherwise, as stated earlier, concentrate on eating "whole foods."

Vitamins

Vitamin A

Benefits:　Vitamin A, a fat-soluble vitamin that stores in the body, is a superantioxidant that is important for immune function, building strong bones, cell division, and more. Liver and eggs contain retinal, a usable form of vitamin A, and colorful fruits and vegetables contain carotenoids that the liver converts to retinal. Beta-carotene is found in many foods.

Getting the proper amount of vitamin A either through animal or plant foods is vital to staying well. Some preliminary studies theorize that vitamin A may be therapeutic to calm the inflammatory response in those with autoimmune diseases, such as rheumatoid arthritis. Contrary to that, other studies show that too much vitamin A can put you at a higher risk for fracture. The study results, published in the January 2002 issue of *The Journal of the American Medical Association*, concluded that women who took supplemental vitamin A were 40 percent more likely to fracture a hip than women who did not. Researchers felt this served as a reminder to everyone that vitamin supplements are not without serious side effects, and reiterates what I have said previously: the best source of vitamins and nutrition is whole foods.

Recommended Daily Intake (RDI):　5,000 International Units (I.U.s) daily. Vitamin A is also measured in retinal equivalents (REs). One RE equals 3.33 I.U.s of retinal (active vitamin A) equals 10 I.U.s of beta-carotene. Do not exceed 8,000 to 10,000 International Units daily from diet and supplements, as vitamin A is toxic in higher doses.

Best food sources: beef and chicken liver, whole milk, cheese, and eggs. You get vitamin A from beta-carotene in carrots, mango, sweet potato, spinach, cantaloupe, kale, apricots, red pepper, broccoli, and fortified foods.

Vitamin C (Ascorbic Acid)

Benefits: Vitamin C, a water-soluble vitamin that must be replenished, is not only important to keep your immune system functioning normally, this influential nutrient also helps to maintain the strength of collagen, ligaments, and tendons and can block the effect of inflammatory substances. As vitamin C inhibits the breakdown of cartilage, it may be of help to those suffering from arthritis whose cartilage is often adversely affected. In the Framingham Osteoarthritis Cohort Study, participants with osteoarthritis of the knee who had a higher intake of vitamin C (300–1,000 milligrams per day of ascorbic acid) also had a reduced risk of cartilage loss and disease progression. Researchers found that abnormal capillary fragility improved, as well as improvement of symptoms.

If you suffer with heavy menstrual bleeding from fibroid tumors or endometriosis, vitamin C helps your body absorb iron, a key mineral that must be replaced in most women of childbearing age. This antioxidant is also important for protecting muscle cells from the damage and pain associated with fibromyalgia syndrome.

Recommended Daily Intake (RDI): 75 milligrams. You can get 90 milligrams of vitamin C by eating five servings of fresh fruits and vegetables daily.

Best food sources: Broccoli, cauliflower, peppers, kale, brussels sprouts, cabbage, citrus fruit, melons, asparagus, avocado, kohlrabi, mustard greens, tomato, and watercress.

Vitamin E (Tocopherol)

Benefits: Vitamin E, a fat-soluble vitamin that stores in the body, may influence many different types of pain, according to preliminary research. For instance, some studies show that foods high in vitamin E can reduce PMS-related breast tenderness, nervousness, depression, headache, fatigue, and insomnia. In a study published in the January 2001 issue of the *British Journal of Obstetrics and Gynaecology*, researchers found that vitamin E could ease menstrual cramps by blocking formulation of prostaglandins (the hormonelike substances implicated in painful menstruation). Studies also confirm that women with fibrocystic breast changes reported relief from breast pain after ingesting vitamin E.

Vitamin E also fights arthritislike damage—in mice. French scientists discovered that vitamin E reduces joint destruction in mice with a rheumatoidlike arthritis. After six weeks of vitamin E treatment, the arthritic mice had less severe bone and cartilage destruction than animals that did not receive vitamin E. In humans, experts believe that rheumatoid arthritis patients have low blood levels of antioxidants, such as vitamin E and C, which are necessary to fight the destructive effects of free radicals, potentially damaging by-products of the body's metabolism.

Recommended Daily Intake (RDI):   30 International Units (IU). The health risk of too much vitamin E supplementation is low, although there are a few studies on long-term supplementation. The Institute of Medicine has set the upper tolerable limit for vitamin E supplementation at 1,500 International Units (1,000 milligrams), as bleeding may occur at higher levels.

Best food sources: Cold-pressed seed oils, wheat germ, nuts, seeds, mango, pumpkin, and green leafy vegetables like broccoli, chard, kohlrabi, spinach, and greens of dandelion, mustard and turnip. You can also find vitamin E in meat, fish, poultry, clams, and shrimp.

Vitamin B1 (Thiamin)

Benefits: Vitamin B1, a water-soluble vitamin, is crucial to convert fats, carbohydrates, and amino acids to energy. While there is no guaranteed link between vitamin B1 and chronic pain, a study published in 2001 in *Cochrane Database of Systematic Reviews,* concluded that 100 milligrams of vitamin B1 taken daily is an effective treatment for painful menstrual cramps.

Recommended Daily Intake   (RDI): 1.5 milligrams for women.

Best food sources: Pork, organ and red meats, whole and enriched grains, nuts, green and deep orange fruits and vegetables, beans, peas, and diary products.

Vitamin B2 (Riboflavin)

Benefits: For migraine headache sufferers, riboflavin may help bring relief. In several controlled studies, this water-soluble B vitamin was shown to reduce the severity and the frequency of migraines.

Riboflavin may bring relief to those with carpal tunnel syndrome by reducing the tingling and numbness in the fingers and keeping the nerves healthy.

Recommended Daily Intake (RDI): 1.7 milligrams daily for women.

Best food sources: Dairy products, green leafy vegetables, whole grain products, baking flour, yeast, and cereals.

Vitamin B3 (Niacin)

Benefits: Vitamin B3 is a water-soluble vitamin, meaning it is not stored in the body and has to be constantly replenished. It comes in two basic forms: niacin (also called nicotinic acid) and niacinamide (also called nicotinamide). Some new National Institute of Health research has linked vitamin B3 with improved joint range of motion and reduced pain and swelling. A study published in October 1999 in *Medical Hypothesis*, researchers concluded that nontoxic nutritional therapies, such as niacinamide, may prove beneficial in preventing and halting osteoarthritis by enhancing glucocorticoid secretion.

Some researchers have used therapeutic doses of vitamin B3 (150 milligrams) as prophylactic treatment for migraine headache with good results. Yet, higher doses (more than 75 milligrams) can cause uncomfortable symptoms, such as flushing, and liver damage may occur.

Recommended Daily Intake (RDI): 20 milligrams.

Best food sources: Brewer's yeast, wheat germ, enriched breads, mushrooms, green vegetables, peanut butter, potatoes, and rice.

Vitamin B6 (Pyridoxine)

Benefits: Vitamin B6 is important for the synthesis of serotonin and dopamine, neurotransmitters that are necessary for healthy nerve cell communication. There are studies in progress on the relationship between vitamin B6 and chronic pain and headache. In fact, those who suffer with migraine headaches often have lower levels of serotonin.

When it comes to easing PMS symptoms, such as bloating, cramping, and irritability, as well as the discomfort from fibrocystic breast changes, vitamin B6 appears to have some therapeutic benefit. Some studies have shown that vitamin B6 increases the accumulation of magnesium within the cells of the body. When paired with foods high in magnesium, foods containing B6 can reduce vulnerability to mood changes during the menstrual cycle.

Several studies suggest that vitamin B6 deficiency may cause an increased susceptibility to carpal tunnel pain and numbness.

Recommended Daily Intake (RDI):   2.0 milligrams. In order to avoid vitamin B6 deficiency, make sure to eat foods that contain this important nutrient on a daily basis. If you do supplement, the Institute of Medicine recently established 100 milligrams of vitamin B6 as the upper limit. Taking too much vitamin B6 may cause nerve damage to the arms and legs.

Best food sources: Chicken, fish, liver, kidney, pork, bananas, spinach, sweet potato, white potato, garbanzo beans, walnuts, brown rice, soybeans, sunflower seeds, avocado, oats, peanuts, lima beans, peanut butter, prunes, and whole wheat products. Fortified cereal has 100 percent of the RDA of vitamin B6, and one banana and one-half cup garbanzo beans give you more than the RDA of vitamin B6.

Folic Acid

Benefits: Folic acid and folate are forms of the water-soluble B vitamin. Folate occurs naturally in food. Folic acid is the synthetic form found in fortified foods and dietary supplements. All women should make sure they get the recommended amount of folate, as it clearly influences many body functions, including the production and maintenance of new cells. Some studies have found that a deficiency in folate can lead to compromised bone, as high levels of homocysteine is thought to play a role in osteoporosis, and folate helps regulate homocysteine. A clinical study among postmenopausal women suggests that folic acid supplementation reduced homocysteine levels, even though none of the women appeared to be deficient in folic acid.

In a study published in the July 2001 issue of *Arthritis and Rheumatism*, researchers confirmed that taking folic acid or folate supplements along with methotrexate, a commonly prescribed medication for rheumatoid arthritis, can help decrease drug-related liver damage. This allows patients to stay on the medication longer and see greater relief of pain and inflammation. Dietary folate may give the same benefit.

Another reason to get ample folate, through food or supplementation, is to improve your mood. Research shows there is a high incidence of folate deficiency in depression, and clinical studies indicate that some depressed patients who are folate deficient respond to folate administration.

Recommended Daily Intake (RDI): 400 micrograms (mcg). If you need to supplement, the risk of toxicity is low.

Best food sources: Fortified breakfast cereals, wheat germ, spinach, oranges, broccoli, asparagus, beets, spinach, turnip greens, cabbage, egg yolks, turkey, cowpeas, chickpeas, lentils, black beans, kidney beans, and soybeans.

Pantothenic Acid

Benefits: Research suggests that people with rheumatoid arthritis may be partially deficient in pantothenic acid, a water-soluble vitamin. In one placebo-controlled trial, patients who took 2,000 milligrams of pantothenic acid per day had less morning stiffness, disability, and pain.

Recommended Daily Intake (RDI): 10 milligrams. While many doctors suggest therapeutic doses of pantothenic acid (sometimes as high as 2,000 milligrams for those with rheumatoid arthritis), the studies are not conclusive. Stick with a daily multivitamin/mineral tablet to ensure getting adequate amounts of pantothenic acid, along with other necessary nutrients.

Best food sources: Brewer's yeast, whole grain breads and cereals, dried beans, avocados, fish, chicken, liver, nuts (pecans, hazelnuts), peanuts, cauliflower, mushrooms, potatoes, oranges, bananas, milk, cheese, and eggs.

B PAIN-FREE

Vitamin	*Food Sources*
B1 (Thiamine)	Wheat germ, peanuts, peas
B2 (Riboflavin)	Dairy products, broccoli, tuna, salmon
B3 (Niacin)	Brewer's yeast, poultry, eggs, peanuts
B6 (Pyridoxine)	Soybeans, liver, fish, bananas, oatmeal
Folic acid	Green leafy vegetables, beans, sweet potatoes, oranges
Pantothenic acid	Cheese, cauliflower, beans, sweet potatoes

Vitamin D

Benefits: Vitamin D (calciferol) is a fat-soluble vitamin and is necessary for your body to absorb calcium from food or supplements.
Along with calcium, vitamin D plays a critical role in maintaining
bone density. While calcium metabolism in the body is dependent
on vitamin D, this vitamin also plays a role in the normal turnover of
articular cartilage. In a study of 556 participants in the Framingham
study, low dietary intake of vitamin D and low serum levels of the
vitamin were each associated with increased progression of
osteoarthritis of the knee. This study suggests adequate intake of
vitamin may slow the progression and possibly help prevent the
development of osteoarthritis.

Vitamin D has similar actions to a hormone in the body as it
helps activate calcium and phosphorus into the bloodstream. Not
only are these two minerals necessary for strong bones, they are also
important in keeping muscles and nerves healthy. When the body
has an insufficient supply of vitamin D, the blood levels of calcium
and phosphorus drop as well. Where does the body turn to get more
of these much-needed minerals? You guessed it: your bones. Loss of
calcium and phosphorus is directly related to osteoporosis and a host
of other bone-weakening problems.

Recommended Daily Intake (RDI):   400 International Units. If
you are over fifty, talk with your doctor about the need for vitamin D
supplements, as the need for this vitamin increases with age. There
is a health risk from taking too much vitamin D, so stay within the
recommended limit.

Best food sources: Halibut-liver oil, herring, cod-liver oil, mackerel, salmon, sardines canned in oil, tuna, fortified milk products,
and fortified cereals.

AN EXTRA BENEFIT FROM YOUR DAILY OUTDOOR WALK

Taking a fifteen- to twenty-minute walk several times a week should
keep your body well supplied with enough vitamin D to keep your
bones healthy. Some studies show that because vitamin D is fat-soluble,
it can store in the body. This means that casual exposure to sunlight
(which gives your body Vitamin D) in the summer months may allow
your body to have ample amounts of this vitamin in the winter.

Vitamin K

Benefits: Vitamin K is an essential nutrient in bone mineralization. Low levels of vitamin K have been found in people with osteopororsis-related fractures. In addition, studies indicate that low levels of circulating vitamin K are associated with low bone density.

Recommended Daily Intake (RDI):   80 micrograms for women.

Best food sources: Broccoli and other cruciferous vegetables, canola oil, soybean oil, bran, beef liver, and olive oil.

Minerals

Boron

Benefits: Boron, an essential trace element for plants, has only recently been considered essential for humans. In Australia, where much of the food is grown on soil deficient in this mineral, it is reported that boron supplements were popular as a treatment for osteoarthritis until the government took them off the market as part of a ban on some natural supplements. In an Australian study, twenty people were randomly assigned to receive boron (six milligrams per day) or a placebo for eight weeks. Fifty percent of those patients who took boron experienced improvement compared with only 10 percent of those taking a placebo. Researchers concluded that boron supplementation may be helpful for individuals with osteoarthritis whose diets are low in boron.

Recommended Daily Intake (RDI):   There is no established recommendation for boron intake.

Best food sources: Iron-enriched cereals and breads, fruits, vegetables, legumes (dried beans and peas), dried fruits, leafy greens, nuts, and seeds.

Calcium

Benefits: Calcium builds strong bones and teeth and helps to prevent osteoporosis, which can gradually lead to painful bone fractures and loss of height. About 91 percent of the body's calcium stores are in the bones and teeth; 1 percent is in the soft tissue and blood. If you do not ingest calcium, the body will take the calcium it needs from the body's stores. After a period, you will get osteoporosis because depleted calcium caused the bones to become weak and less dense. Many foods are high in calcium, including soy products, which are also low in fat. For women with PMS, calcium can reduce abdominal cramping and muscular contractions.

Recommended Daily Intake (RDI):   1,000 milligrams; women 51 and older need 1,200 milligrams or more.

Best food sources: Artichokes, broccoli, bok choy, brussel sprouts, cabbage, carrots, celery, lima beans, spinach, swiss chard, salmon, sardines with bones, kale, beans (dried), dairy products, soy products, and calcium-fortified foods.

Calcium Supplements: Also Effective

While I recommend using food sources of calcium, calcium supplements are also effective in boosting the body's source of calcium. In many studies, calcium citrate has been found to dissolve more easily than carbonate or phosphate, and it is bioavailable, meaning your body can use more of what you ingest. If you take calcium supplements, be sure to follow these rules:

- Avoid taking more than 500 milligrams at once.
- Take supplements with food for best absorption.
- Do not take supplements with high-fat or high-fiber foods, as these foods interfere with the absorption of calcium.
- Do not take calcium supplements with foods high in iron.

Iodine

Benefits: Some studies that suggest iodine may protect against fibrocystic breast changes because of an anti-inflammatory effect.

Recommended Daily Intake (RDI):   150 micrograms.

Best food sources: Fresh or saltwater seafood and shellfish, foods grown in iodine-rich soil, milk, and iodized-enriched bread or salt.

Iron

Benefits: Some specific nutritional deficiencies can influence how you feel. For instance, if you are not including iron-rich foods in your diet (especially menstruating women or those who have heavy periods because of fibroid tumors or endometriosis), then iron-deficiency anemia can result. Symptoms of fatigue, weakness, shortness of breath, and pallor can compound the chronic pain symptoms you feel each day.

Recommended Daily Intake (RDI): 18 milligrams.

Best food sources: Dried apricots, dried beans, enriched or fortified breads and cereals, lean red meat (beef, veal, or lamb), lentils, prunes, and raisins. Note: When eating an iron-rich food from a plant source, include a vitamin C source, such as orange or grapefruit juice, along with it to enhance iron absorption.

Magnesium

Benefit: Some researchers believe magnesium holds the key to resolving many types of chronic pain. In the body, magnesium converts vitamin D, which the body needs to take advantage of bone-strengthening calcium, into a form that it can use efficiently. By contributing to increased bone density, the mineral may help stall the onset of osteoporosis.

Some experts find that migraine sufferers are magnesium-deficient, and supplementing with 400 milligrams daily of magnesium oxide or chelated magnesium diminishes the frequency of the migraines as well as reducing the severity of migraine pain. Magnesium also may help to ease tension headaches, muscle cramps, muscle strains, and muscle tension. If you have a magnesium deficiency, you may experience excessive muscle tension, which may trigger muscle spasms, restlessness, tics, and twitches.

If you suffer with fibromyalgia, magnesium appears to inhibit nerve receptors linked to the trigger point pain and to regulate the release of neurohormones. In a study published in the March 2002 issue of *Alternative Medicine Alert*, researchers found that an oral dose of 500 milligrams a day of magnesium significantly increases muscle magnesium level and influences fibromyalgia symptoms. (Side effects of magnesium supplements may include gastrointestinal symptoms and diarrhea.)

In a study published in *Cochrane Database of Systematic Reviews* (2001), researchers found that magnesium supplementation can help alleviate painful menstrual cramps, but they are still unsure how much women might need. Other studies suggest magnesium may help with symptoms of PMS and fibrocystic breast changes. Further research is necessary to determine its effectiveness and the exact dosage required.

Recommended Daily Intake (RDI):   400 milligrams. Dietary magnesium does not present a health risk, but there are risks with taking too much of magnesium supplementation.

Best food sources: Cereals, nuts, sunflower seeds, tofu, diary products, bananas, pineapples, plantains, raisins, artichokes, avocados, lima beans, spinach, okra, beet greens, hummus, oysters, halibut, mackerel, grouper, cod, and sole. You can get magnesium in your daily diet by using various herbs, including coriander, dill, celery seed, sage, dried mustard, basil, cumin, tarragon, marjoram, and poppy seed.

Manganese

Benefits: Manganese is a trace element that is vital for forming connective tissue and building strong bones. In a study published in the February 1999 issue of *Military Medicine*, researchers treated patients with degenerative joint disease of the knee or back using a combination of manganese, glucosamine, and chondroitin. After sixteen weeks, patients with knee osteoarthritis felt improvement from the pain and stiffness. Researchers concluded that adding manganese to the daily supplement therapy may help patients realize a lessening of pain.

Recommended Daily Intake (RDI):   2.0 milligrams. There are almost no cases of manganese deficiency known in humans, and supplementation with manganese could be toxic. Eating a proper diet rich in plant foods is the best way to keep your body supplied with ample amounts of this trace element.

Best food sources: Organ meat, dried beans, leafy vegetables, dried fruit, nuts, unrefined cereals, and whole grains.

Phosphorus

Benefits: Phosphorus and calcium work hand in hand in forming new bone. In individuals whose diets are low in phosphorus, calcium supplementation alone is inadequate and in fact can aggravate an existing phosphorus deficiency. As a result, a calcium phosphate product may be preferable for women undergoing bone-building therapy, according to a study presented recently at the National Osteoporosis Foundation Symposium in Honolulu.

Recommended Daily Intake (RDI):   1,000 milligrams.

Best food sources: Meat, fish, nuts, beans, breads, dairy products, breads, cereals, and other grain products.

Selenium

Benefits: Selenium is a trace mineral that may hold the key to staying disease-free, as it helps keep the immune system working optimally and is important for a healthy thyroid gland. Selenium is an important part of the antioxidant enzyme as it helps to fight free radicals that cause damage to healthy tissue.

Some studies of rheumatoid arthritis patients indicate that they have reduced selenium levels in their blood. Current findings are preliminary, and no recommendations for selenium supplements are available.

Recommended Daily Intake (RDI):   70 micrograms.

Best food sources: Brazil nuts, beef, tuna, turkey, chicken, walnuts, cheese, eggs, cottage cheese, and enriched grain products. One three and one-half-ounce serving of tuna gives you a full day's requirement of selenium.

Zinc

Benefits: Zinc, an essential mineral for good health, keeps your immune system actively fighting viruses and bacteria and helps support healthy growth and development. There is some evidence that the low zinc levels in women prone to PMS indicates that a diet rich in this important mineral may prevent painful PMS symptoms. For osteoporosis prevention, zinc is also crucial as it enhances mineral absorption and is essential for bone health.

Recommended Daily Intake (RDI):   15 milligrams.

Best food sources: Meat, pork, poultry, seafood, wheat products, nuts, seeds, dairy products, and fortified products.

CAFFEINE OR NOT?

While a cup or two of coffee in the morning may increase alertness, in a study published in the October 2001 issue of *Fertility and Sterility,* researchers concluded that drinking more than two cups of coffee a day may boost a woman's estrogen levels and exacerbate endometriosis and fibrocystic breast changes. Caffeine is also thought to increase the symptoms and pain of these problems. However, if you suffer with migraine or tension headaches, that cup of java may ease the pain, as caffeine is often an ingredient in headache medications.

DRINK UP!

Many people ignore the importance of drinking plenty of water each day, and end up dehydrated. Because more than two-thirds of your body weight is water, water is just as important as oxygen for keeping you alive. Imagine every cell, tissue, and organ—all depending on water to function. Water keeps your body alive by stabilizing the temperature, eliminating toxins and waste products, carrying nutrients throughout the body, and maintaining blood volume. Water is also the medium in which cell chemical reactions take place. You could go for weeks without food, but you will live only a few days with no water. Aim for eight or more glasses of water daily, and see if you don't start to feel more energetic and alive.

Super Pain Busters

While I'm helping you focus on food as a natural therapy for easing pain, I want to introduce a few "super foods" that may help. These foods work in various ways to reduce inflammation or bolster the immune system to keep diseases at bay. Select foods from this list, and include them in your daily dietary plan.

Fish

Scientists are now looking at some types of oily fish as having pain-relieving functions. The essential fatty acids in salmon, tuna, and trout, among others, act as anti-inflammatory compounds and may help the body absorb iodine. Low levels of iodine are associated with fibrocystic breast changes. Supplementation with omega-3 fatty acids may also alleviate painful menstrual cramps.

For those with arthritis, the omega-3 fatty acids in fish have an anti-inflammatory effect, which helps reduce swelling and pain in the joints. In a study published in the January 2000 issue of the *American Journal of Clinical Nutrition*, researchers concluded that patients with rheumatoid arthritis who took dietary supplements of omega-3 fatty acids had fewer tender joints and morning stiffness.

Cod liver oil may not be appetizing, but researchers at Cardiff University in Wales have found that this fishy tonic is effective in treating arthritic joint pain and even slowing or reversing the destruction of joint cartilage—good news for women with painful osteoarthritis. Researchers believe that the omega-3 fatty acids in the oil "switch off" the collagen-degrading enzymes that break down joint cartilage. This leads to a slower progression of cartilage destruction, and reduces inflammation and the subsequent pain.

FISH HIGH IN OMEGA-3

Anchovies	Salmon
Bluefish	Sardines
Capelin	Shad
Dogfish	Sturgeon
Herring	Tuna
Mackerel	Whitefish

Super Vegetables

Red Peppers. Capsaicin appears to reduce levels of substance P, the compound in the body that triggers inflammation and pain impulses from the central nervous system. Eating hot red peppers may burn your tongue, but they can also interrupt the pain perception elsewhere in your body. This may be because capsaicin, the pain-relieving chemical in hot red peppers, is thought to trigger the body to release endorphins, nature's own opiates. Red pepper also contains aspirinlike compounds known as salicylates.

Sweet Peppers. Although only preliminary information is available, an ingredient in sweet peppers (capsiate) may possess anti-inflammatory properties that could be beneficial in various chronic inflammatory states (e.g. rheumatoid arthritis and inflammatory bowel disease).

Broccoli. Broccoli contains glutathione, a powerful antioxidant and detoxifying agent. Without glutathione, other antioxidants such as vitamins C and E cannot do their job and protect you adequately against disease. Research indicates that people who are low in this antioxidant are more likely to have arthritis than those who have higher amounts. Other glutathione-rich foods include asparagus, cabbage, cauliflower, potatoes, and tomatoes. Fruits with glutathione include avocados, grapefruit, oranges, peaches, and watermelon.

Celery. There are some indications that celery helps to reduce uric acid in the body—the trigger of gouty arthritis. It also has about twenty-four other anti-inflammatory compounds, including a substance called apigenin, which has an aspirinlike effect in the body.

Less Decaf Coffee and More Tea

According to research presented at the American College of Rheumatology Annual Scientific Meeting (2001), older women should stay away from decaf coffee to diminish the risk of developing rheumatoid arthritis. Researchers following the participants in the Iowa Women's Health Study, found that women who drank four or more cups of decaffeinated coffee daily were more than twice as likely to develop rheumatoid arthritis during the course of follow-up. In contrast, those women who drank large amounts of tea, more than three cups daily, had a 60 percent reduced risk in developing rheumatoid arthritis.

In another study, presented at the Society of Critical Care Medicine, researchers found that green tea may help block the arthritis-inflammatory response. Green tea contains a type of polyphenol known as epigallocatechin-3-gallate, or EGCG, that inhibits the expression of the interleukin-8 gene, which is a substance that signals the body's white blood cells and other mediators to promote inflammation. Researchers theorize that "more may be better" when it comes to drinking green tea to help reduce pain and stiffness.

Super Fruits

Pineapple.   For years, coaches have recommended pineapple to athletes to help heal sports injuries. The reason is bromelain, the key enzyme in pineapple that helps reduce inflammation. For women with carpal tunnel syndrome, there are some findings that eating pineapple may help to reduce tissue swelling. Likewise, a German study found bromelain enzymes resulted in a statistical reduction of pain in patients with knee osteoarthritis, as well as those with rheumatoid arthritis.

Citrus Fruits.   Citrus fruits such as oranges and grapefruits may give you a double whammy against pain. Not only are these juicy fruits filled with vitamin C (ascorbic acid), they are high in bioflavonoids. Bioflavonoids come from plants and have strong antioxidant and anti-inflammatory properties.

Blueberries. Dark berries (blueberries, blackberries, cherries, and raspberries) are helpful in easing pain because they contain anthocyanidins, which help to stabilize the collagen found in bones. Cherries help to lower uric acid in the body and prevent gouty arthritis attacks.

Soy

A diet high in soy products may be the answer for chronic pain sufferers in the not-too-distant future. Some researchers from Johns Hopkins have found that rats on a soy-based diet experienced "significantly less" swelling and were able to tolerate more pain than the test group given a milk protein.

New studies also show that adding one serving a day of soybeans may actually increase bone strength. A recent study was conducted at the University of Illinois on sixty-six postmenopausal women who were not taking hormone replacement therapy. Of this group, the women who took in 90 milligrams of isoflavones (the phytoestrogen found in soy foods) daily for six months increased their bone density by *3 percent*, as well as the bone mineral content of the lumbar spine. (The lumbar spine, at the small of the back, is prone to fractures after menopause.) While the increase was small, it is extremely significant and offers tremendous hope to women who choose not to take estrogen replacement therapy at menopause.

In osteoporosis research, the isoflavones genistein and daidzein, two components of the soybean, are thought to inhibit bone breakdown in animals because of their estrogenlike actions. Studies show that eating animal protein can weaken bones, as it causes the body to remove calcium more quickly. In a breakthrough study, researchers found that those who ate soy protein instead of animal protein lost *50 percent less* calcium in the urine, thus helping to keep bones dense and strong. Because some Japanese women have half the rate of hip fractures as women in the United States, preliminary studies suggest that not only does soy help in blocking cancer and heart disease, but it may be the key factor in helping to retain bone mass.

SIMPLE SOY SOLUTIONS

Here are a few of the many easy and appetizing ways you can incorporate soy in your diet:

- Use silken tofu in desserts like tofu shakes, puddings, and in creamy soups.
- Use textured vegetable protein to replace ground beef. Saute with favorite herbs and spices and toss in spaghetti sauce, chili, tacos, or sloppy Joe sandwiches.
- Substitute tofu or miso for cream cheese when making dips. Blend with chopped vegetables, spices, or prepackaged dip mixes.
- Use soy cheeses as toppings for pizza or as cheese substitutes in pasta recipes.
- Use soymilk as a dairy substitute in smoothies, cream-based sauces, and soups.
- Use miso to flavor soups, sauces, and marinades.
- Toss miso into a vegetarian stir fry to give more flavor.
- Use soymilk instead of dairy for puddings, sauces, and pie fillings.
- Pour soymilk over hot and cold cereals, and use in coffee or tea instead of cream.
- Sprinkle soy granules on cereal, yogurt, or ice cream.
- Add soy granules to meatloaf, stews, casseroles, and baked goods.
- Grill tempeh, coat with barbeque sauce, and serve on a bun.
- Use a quarter cup of isolated soy protein powder with every cup of ricotta cheese when making pasta dishes.
- Make egg salad using firm tofu as a replacement for chopped eggs.

CHAPTER FOURTEEN

Step 6: Reduce Pain with Mind/Body Exercises

When Liz feels a migraine headache coming on, she drops whatever she's doing at the time, turns on her favorite John Coltrane CD, and starts a series of relaxation exercises. If she's at home, her three children know to leave her alone for thirty minutes. When she's at work, her administrative assistant holds all calls until Liz has finished her relaxation therapy. This thirty-nine-year-old CPA claims to stop most migraines in their tracks, catching the first symptom before it escalates by using a series of mind/body techniques to de-stress.

Learning to relax in the midst of interminable pain is not an easy skill. Nevertheless, Liz has learned to bring about the relaxation response at will whenever she feels the first sign of tension in her temples and brow.

I admire what Liz and other women have learned as they use mind/body exercises to remove themselves mentally and emotionally from the painful moment. The problem with pain is that it's multifaceted and extremely complex. Not only is it influenced by physiological events; there are also psychological, social, and spiritual elements to it. Pain is not like an infected throat, where you can take an antibiotic, and in a few days, there's no more pain. You cannot put an ointment on pain, hoping it will never return. Many times, your doctor cannot even find what's causing the pain. Unlike a fracture or a known disease, soft-tissue pain may not appear on an X ray or even respond to medical treatment. Moreover, how do you measure pain? What may be horrible pain to one woman is considered mild by another.

Because pain is so elusive and difficult to measure, it lends itself well to complementary therapies. In that regard, mind/body interventions can let you become the master of your pain. In a study published in the May 2, 2001 issue of *The Journal of the American Medical Association*, researchers concluded that relaxation therapies could decrease pain when used in conjunction with medications. In this study, researchers found that when patients take pain medications for a long time, the body adjusts to that level of medication. However, when participants used stress management and relaxation therapies along with pain medication, they reported having fewer headaches and took less of the pain relievers. In fact, patients who used medications, in this case antidepressants, along with relaxation therapies were able to discontinue their medications after one year, compared with patients who took medication alone. While unsure as to why relaxation exercises work to decrease pain, the researchers believed that muscle relaxation and stretching might reduce the number of pain signals delivered to the nervous system.

"Can my innermost thoughts really affect the pain I feel?" you might ask. Definitely! An intriguing school of medicine called psychoneuroimmunology, or the study of mind/body interplay, is based on the premise that mental or emotional processes (the mind) affect physiologic function (the body). Health professionals in this field estimate that between 90 and 95 percent of all health problems can be traced to a contributing influence of emotions. Some are going so far as to say that an optimistic outlook, such as a feeling of control, may in some way protect against disease or illness and act as a valuable complement to conventional medical care.

Yet, when you live with chronic pain for months or years, you certainly can feel "loss of control," which can lead to a constant state of tension that intensifies your pain. Whether from kids, carpools, or career pressure, you know how the slightest bit of daily stress can cause your pain to intensify. Perhaps coping with a rambunctious toddler causes your migraine pain to be more frequent. Dealing with impetuous clients at work may cause your lower back to ache. One of my patients, Ginah, a successful book editor at a large publishing house in New York, suffers with chronic neck and back pain because of a previous injury. This forty-two-year-old woman said that when her days are smooth and she can do her job without interruption, she hardly feels any pain. But on days when her writers forget important deadlines or copy editors miss manuscript errors, the back of Ginah's neck and her shoulders begin to throb. She said it's as if her neck and shoulders have a mind of their own and react to her stressors with excruciating pain.

So this step is very important in your program to end pain. I'm going to discuss some specific mind/body tools that can help you to take control of your body's reaction to stress and finally learn to relax. For example, the relaxation response, discussed below, helps you *reduce* physical stress and negative thoughts and *increase* your inner ability to self-manage pain. Biofeedback, another mind/body tool, alerts you to stress symptoms before they cause injury to your body. Listening to soothing music reduces pain by interrupting the cycle of pain, muscle tension, and sympathetic activity. Other therapies help divert your attention, and distraction is an essential part of living with chronic pain. Each of these benefits has a positive effect on your well-being and your outlook on life.

Find the mind/body technique that works best for you. You may have to try each of these to see which one has a good "fit" with your daily schedule and type of pain. Then, as you select the therapies that give you the greatest benefit, be sure to use them daily, as they become a part of your more relaxed lifestyle.

WHAT TRIGGERS YOUR PAIN?

Daily stress often makes pain accelerate. This stress could be environmental or internal, caused by any of the following:

- A telephone ringing nonstop
- Relatives coming for dinner
- Waiting in the doctor's office for an appointment
- Standing in line at the store
- An unexpected bill in the mail
- Being put on hold when speaking with a friend
- Buying a home
- Unexpected home repairs
- Telephone solicitors
- A neighbor's barking dog at night

Relaxation Response

The relaxation response came from the concentrated research of Dr. Herbert Benson, author of *The Relaxation Response* and founder of the Mind/Body Medical Institute at Harvard University. Benson was the first medical doctor to scientifically document the physiological benefits of meditation through his studies with experienced Transcendental Meditators. As one of the great pioneers of mind/body medicine, Benson helps explain PNI (psychoneurology immunology), of mind/body interplay, suggesting that the practice of medicine is like a three-legged stool, where the legs of surgery and medications are balanced with spiritual self-care. This means that while medical science is crucial for keeping us well, the mind/body connection may be equally important in staving off illness altogether.

The relaxation response actually changes the physical and emotional responses to stress. For instance, when you elicit the relaxation response, you'll notice a visible decrease in your heart rate, blood pressure, and muscle tension. Recent studies have found that relaxation therapy appears to produce improved adjustment, increased medication compliance, and decreased use of medical services for those with chronic pain. Imagine the benefit of using this mind/body therapy when you're stuck in a traffic jam with a car full of active kids, or sitting at an all-day business conference, especially if stress triggers your pain. Once you master the technique of relaxing your body, you can go from stressed to de-stressed in a matter of minutes.

Meditative techniques are also a key element in the Arthritis Self-help Course at Stanford University. More than 100,000 people with arthritis have taken the twelve-hour course and learned meditation-style relaxation exercises as part of a comprehensive self-care program. Graduates report a 15 to 20 percent reduction in pain.

Basic Instructions for the Relaxation Response

As you learn mind/body therapies, set aside a period of about twenty minutes each day that you can devote to relaxation practice. Go to a quiet room where you will not be disturbed. It's a good idea to turn off your phone for this session, and close your door. Remove any outside distractions that could disrupt your concentration. Recline comfortably on a rug, bed, or couch, supporting your entire body so you do not feel added muscle tension or unnecessary pain. Use a pillow or cushion under your head if this helps.

During the twenty-minute relaxation period, remain perfectly still. Be mindful of your thoughts at that moment and try to block intruding thoughts, such as your upcoming schedule or what you are planning for dinner. Imagine that every muscle in your body is becoming loose, relaxed, and free of any excess tension. Focus on your breathing as you relax your muscles; try to breathe slowly and rhythmically. As you exhale, imagine all your muscles becoming more relaxed, as if you are breathing your pain away.

At the end of twenty minutes, try to focus on what this relaxed state feels like. Do your muscles feel tight or relaxed? Is your mind at peace, or still concerned with all you must do that day? Focusing on your relaxed state will help you remember how it feels so your body and mind can learn to mimic this again.

Don't be surprised if the relaxed feeling you achieve begins to fade and dissipate once you get up and return to your normal activities. Many women find that it is only after several weeks of daily, consistent practice that they are able to maintain the relaxed feeling beyond the practice session itself. However, if practiced regularly, your body will soon learn to elicit the relaxation response and target the sympathetic nervous system, which is linked to your skin, blood vessels, and organs. This, in turn, will help to relieve any anxiety that often accompanies chronic pain.

Deep Abdominal Breathing

An old proverb states, "Life is in the breath. He who half breathes, half lives." Breathing is one of the few activities of the body that we can consciously control. *Pranayama*, which is the conscious focus on and control of breath to heal disease, is an important part of ancient yoga. In fact, before you learn any of the yoga postures, the instructor will teach you how to breathe properly.

Breathing is also important in alleviating childbirth pain. For years, women have practiced slow, patterned breathing techniques to help keep them focused on labor. This deep abdominal breathing actually alters your psychological state, making a painful moment diminish in intensity. Think how your respiration quickens when your pain intensifies. Then consider how taking a deep, slow breath brings an immediate calming effect, reducing both anxiety and level of pain. If you measured your heart rate at a time when you were completely overwhelmed with stress, and then measured it again after doing ten minutes of deep abdominal breathing, you'd be convinced of the physiological transformation that takes place.

Researchers know that the brain makes its own morphinelike pain relievers, called *endorphins* and *enkephalins.* These hormones are associated with a happy, positive feeling and can help pain messages from reaching the brain. During deep abdominal breathing, you will add oxygen to the blood and cause your body to release endorphins, while decreasing the release of stress hormones and slowing down your heart rate.

Basic Instructions for Deep Abdominal Breathing

Go to a quiet room where there are no distractions. Let your family members know you are taking a time-out, so they do not disturb you. Take the phone off the hook, and close the door. Lie comfortably on your back, and place your hands on your abdomen. Close your eyes, calm your racing mind, and then take in a slow, deliberate, deep breath, counting to five as you do so. Make sure your hands rise, so you know your abdomen is expanding. If your hands do not rise, yet you see your chest rising, you are breathing incorrectly. Try again. When you are breathing correctly, inhale to a count of five, pause for three seconds, and then exhale to a count of five. Start with ten repetitions of this exercise, and then increase to twenty-five.

You might find deep abdominal breathing helpful when you are experiencing increased pain and are waiting for your pain medications to kick in. The slow deep breathing can interrupt a cycle of rapid, shallow breathing and result in a more comfortable state of mind.

Progressive Muscle Relaxation

Many women who suffer with chronic pain are unaware of the enormous amount of tension they hold in their bodies. Take Mindy, for example. This forty-one-year-old teacher suffered for years with fibromyalgia, including chronic deep muscle pain and unrelenting fatigue. While Mindy didn't think she was tightening her muscles under stress, she became aware once she learned progressive muscle relaxation, that she had been contributing to much of her constant muscle tension. For instance, after a long day of teaching thirty second-graders, Mindy's neck and shoulder muscles were hard and tight. Using progressive muscle relaxation, she realized that she could greatly reduce this tension by recognizing what muscle tightness felt like and then intentionally reducing the increased pressure.

Basic Instructions for Progressive Muscle Relaxation

This mind/body technique involves contracting, then relaxing, all the different muscle groups in the body, beginning with your head and neck and progressing down to your arms, chest, back, stomach, pelvis, legs, and feet.

Practice this exercise during your daily time-out period. Lie down on a bed or rug in a quiet room with no distractions. Starting from the top or bottom of your body, focus on each set of your muscles. Tense the muscles to the count of ten, then release to the count of ten. Go slowly as you progress throughout your body, taking as long as you can. Get in touch with each part and feel the tension you are experiencing. Also, notice how it feels to be tension-free as you release the muscle. It's important to do progressive muscle relaxation in combination with deep abdominal breathing: breathe in while tensing the muscles; breathe out or exhale while relaxing them.

Studies show that when you can create a strong mental image using this type of relaxation technique, you actually feel "removed" from the pain you feel. This *mindfulness*, or focusing all attention on what you feel at the moment, can help you move beyond the pain as you become centered in a world of health and inner healing.

Visualization (Guided Imagery)

Visualization, or guided imagery, is another mind/body tool that has helped many women control emotional distress, anxiety, and pain. While some women seem to be naturally better at imagining than others, this simple technique is one that anyone can learn.

Basic Instructions for Visualization

Take a time-out in a quiet surrounding without distractions. You can sit in a comfortable chair, lie down, or even sit outdoors and enjoy the peacefulness of nature. During this time, try to visualize or imagine a calm, relaxing scene. This might be a retreat spot you have enjoyed at the seashore or by a lake in the mountains. Focus on this relaxing place, and attempt to recapture the moment as you envision the sounds, smells, textures, and feelings you would experience at that place. Become aware of your breathing and anxiety level as you focus, and do not let any outside stimulus disrupt your imagery time.

Music Therapy

Perhaps the most popular relaxation modality is music therapy. Whether New Age, rock, jazz, or classical, many women find that music distracts them from the painful moment, helping to reduce mental stress. In fact, in some hospitals, staff members give patients tapes of soothing music and reassuring voice-overs to use during surgical procedures. In clinical studies, both doctors and patients agreed that listening to music produced greater decreases in peaks of tension, and produced greater compliance with relaxation practice. While the studies are limited, it's thought that music therapy can help to improve mood and pain tolerance. This therapy is thought to enhance the parasympathetic response through the effects of sound, encouraging relaxation at a deep level.

Basic Instructions for Music Therapy

If you listen to music for relaxation and pain reduction, avoid melodies that make you feel tense or that cause uneasiness. Allow time each day to listen to your favorite relaxation music, and use this with another mind/body therapy, such as visualization or deep abdominal breathing. Make sure that the pace of the music you choose is slower than your heart rate, or approximately 60 beats a minute, as this can slow down a racing heart rate. Some studies have shown that music can lower blood pressure and boost your immune cell count while reducing levels of stress hormones. Reduced stress will result in less pain.

Spirituality

There are many new studies on the relationship of spirituality to chronic pain illnesses. Researchers in the field of psychoneuroim-munology report growing evidence on the positive effects of spirituality, contending that the human body has a powerful sacramental dimension to it, and those who acknowledge this with a strong sense of higher purpose—a body-soul connectedness—are the ones who are more likely to stay with programs that lead to optimal health. This does not mean that belief in God or a Higher Power should replace medicine. However, faith in something greater than yourself offers a type of curative power, helping you disconnect unhealthy worries and replace them with soothing belief.

According to the latest medical research, religious faith is healthy and even healing. Studies show that prayer and meditation produce alpha and theta waves in the brain that are consistent with serenity and happiness, allowing your harried thoughts to have a reprieve. In a study done at Johns Hopkins School of Medicine on women with rheumatoid arthritis, researchers concluded that spirituality might be a type of psychological resource that allows individuals to adjust better to living with a chronic illness. They found that those who had a high level of spirituality and were more likely to attend church and pray rated themselves as healthier and less disabled than their less spiritual peers.

In a study published in the December 2000 issue of the *Journal of Holistic Nursing*, researchers from the University of Florida and Wayne State University found that most older adults use prayer more than any other alternative health remedy to help manage the stress in their lives. In addition, nurse researchers found that prayer is the most frequently reported alternative treatment used by seniors to feel better or maintain health in general. In the report, 96 percent of older adults use prayer to specifically cope with stress, and 84 percent of the respondents reported using prayer more than other alternative remedies to feel better or to maintain their health.

In another study published in the April 2001 issue of *The Journal of Pain*, researchers found that patients who were able to control and decrease pain with spiritual coping strategies were less likely to experience joint pain. These religious patients also had moods that were more positive, higher levels of social support, and positive coping skills.

Biofeedback

Biofeedback is a mind/body relaxation technique that uses electronics to measure such stress-related body responses as heart rate or muscle contractions. This type of therapy is based on the idea that when people are given information about their body's internal processes, they can use this information to learn to control those processes. There is good evidence that biofeedback might help relieve many types of chronic pain, including tension and migraine headaches, according to a consensus statement from the National Institutes of Health. In one study by researchers at the Department of Psychology, University of South Alabama, 80 percent of children who suffered with migraines were symptom-free after receiving intensive biofeedback training. In other research, some headache patients who were able to increase hand temperature using thermal biofeedback also experienced fewer and less intense migraine headaches.

With biofeedback, you are connected to a machine that informs you and your therapist when you are physically relaxing your body. With sensors placed over specific muscle sites, the therapist will read the tension in your muscles, heart rate, breathing pattern, the amount of sweat produced, or body temperature. Any or all of these readings can let the trained biofeedback therapist know if you are learning to relax. Because the instruments magnify signals that you might not otherwise notice, you can use this visual or auditory response to learn how to control certain bodily functions.

The ultimate goal of biofeedback is to use this skill outside the therapist's office when you are facing real stressors. For those with chronic pain, you know the real stressor is pain itself. Nevertheless, other daily stressors can cause your pain to flare. Learning to respond in a healthy way to the chronic stressors is the goal. If learned properly, electronic biofeedback can help you control your heart rate, blood pressure, breathing patterns, and muscle tension when you are *not* hooked up to the machine.

The following are some of the common types of biofeedback:

- Electromyographic (EMG) biofeedback provides feedback on muscle tension and works well for patients with anxiety disorders or chronic pain.
- Electrodermal (EDR) measures subtle changes in amounts of perspiration.
- Thermal biofeedback is used in teaching hand warming. This has been found to help relieve migraine headaches and can benefit people with Raynaud's disease, a disorder that causes the blood vessels in the fingers, toes, ears, and nose to constrict (narrow).

- Finger pulse biofeedback records heart rate and force and is useful for anxiety or cardiovascular symptoms.
- Respiration feedback shows the rate, volume, rhythm, and location of each breath.

Hypnosis

Hypnosis is another alternative tool used to control stress and postoperative pain. Although hypnosis comes from the Greek word meaning "sleep," it is really an intense state of focused concentration or imagination. While this is not a new mind/body method of treatment, it is now being used in innovative ways to improve the quality of care after surgery.

Hypnosis is substantiated in scientific research, and several new studies confirm that the power of hypnosis can help reduce pain, anxiety, and blood pressure in patients undergoing invasive medical procedures. One study published in the April 2000 issue of the journal *The Lancet* reported that medical procedures took significantly less time in the hypnosis treatment group (as opposed to the group that received positive affirmation and encouragement), and patients in the hypnosis group took less than half as much painkilling medication as the standard group.

If done correctly, hypnosis can produce a feeling of calm and improve your confidence in handling pain. Some women even feel a dramatic difference with less pain after a session. While experts are unsure exactly how hypnosis works, many believe it actually alters or changes the brain wave patterns, similar to relaxation therapies. Because hypnosis is not meant for everyone, you should seek a qualified clinical psychologist or psychiatrist to decide if it would work for you.

The Role of Psychotherapy

When chronic pain makes it difficult to cope with everyday issues, you may want to consider behavior interventions and seek therapy with a licensed mental health counselor. Remember, pain not only affects how you feel, it can also influence your emotional state, leaving you anxious, fearful, and even depressed. Behavior medicine specialists who deal exclusively or largely with chronic pain are preferable and may offer other alternatives, including cognitive behavioral techniques, which can be implemented in your daily routine.

With psychotherapy in pain management, you voice any pent-up emotions with a trained therapist and then begin to learn some appropriate coping strategies to deal with these issues. In most cases, it is important that your therapist is familiar with the dynamics of chronic pain. You may opt for individual counseling, family counseling, or even group counseling where you can talk with others who suffer with chronic pain.

Some women find support groups extremely helpful as they can express their feelings about a "life with pain," and receive comfort and encouragement from others. Knowing that someone else identifies with what you are going through helps you feel validated.

Support groups are not meant to be professional therapy groups. Those who would benefit from standard psychological or psychiatric intervention should seek professional treatment to fit their needs.

Laughter

Laughter may potentially relax tense muscles, reduce heart rate and blood pressure, exercise the muscles of the face, diaphragm, and abdomen, boost the immune system, and lead to the release of endorphins (the body's own pain-fighting hormones). Researchers have shown that muscle tension may remain low for up to 45 minutes after a period of vigorous laughter—real belly laughter can relax the muscles more than a vigorous massage.

Be Your Own Pain Expert

Because chronic pain lingers for months or even years, it's important to become your own bodyguard—and be your own pain expert. You can learn to make decisions that will help you de-stress your body and lessen pain, allowing you to reduce pain medications and increase normal activities. It is vital to communicate with your doctor and talk openly about alternative therapies, in case you might have some limitations. Working with your doctor, you can find an acceptable and risk-free way to blend the conventional with the alternative.

Again, be openly discriminating when choosing your mind/body therapies. Just because something is "natural" does not mean it is safe. With your doctor's approval, use the therapies that will boost your inner healing and help move you on the road to wellness and an active life.

CHAPTER FIFTEEN

Step 7: Try Bodywork, Massage, and Other Hands-on Therapies

I watched Maureen massage her temples as she described her long-time battle with tension headaches. This forty-seven-year-old attorney from Boston was in obvious pain when we first started talking, but it seemed that the longer she gently rubbed her forehead, the more relaxed and calm she became.

What's the first thing you do when your head begins to pound or your back begins to ache? If you're like Maureen and many other women, you immediately touch the painful site. For whatever reason, humans seem to have this innate need to rub, massage, or press the body at the first sign of discomfort.

Today we have come a long way in understanding the importance of healing touch. For instance, researchers have reported decreased cortisol and increased numbers and activity of natural killer cell activity following massage therapy. (Natural killer cells are immune system cells that are important in killing virus-infected cells and cancer cells.) Some researchers believe that massage or hands-on therapies might increase the body's natural production of the brain chemical serotonin, which is associated with pain-relieving effects. We know that massage therapy improves blood circulation, speeds healing, and lowers the stress hormones cortisol and norepinephrine, which is thought to diminish their deleterious effect on the immune system. A relaxing massage can also lower blood pressure and heart rate.

Nonetheless, whether or not healing touch causes physiological changes in the body, it simply feels good to be touched. A deep muscle massage can alleviate back pain and make you feel renewed; firm pressure on an aching joint can help stop the throbbing pain. That's why I believe touch therapies to be an important part of a woman's plan to end pain. Let's look at some of the most common touch therapies, starting with those that have ancient roots, to see how touch can help you manage your chronic pain.

Asian Medical Therapies

Many historians speculate that massage or touch therapies began as a medical treatment in China. The ancient Chinese medicine practitioners believed that when the body was in balance between yin and yang, health was predominant, and when the yin and yang were imbalanced, disease occurred. Today Chinese medicine practitioners view yin and yang as a way of seeing life—that all things work together to be part of a whole; nothing is seen in isolation or as absolute. This attitude is contrary to Western medicine, where doctors may treat a specific illness alone without taking into consideration the overall health of the person's mind, body, and spirit.

Acupressure Triggers the Release of Endorphins

Acupressure was one of the first healing touch therapies in ancient China and was used before acupuncture. While it uses the same bodily points, there are no needles. This popular form of Chinese healing uses touch to unblock Qi (pronounced "chee"), life energy that is vital to one's health, and to allow the meridians or pathways to flow smoothly. In Oriental medicine, Qi travels along twelve imaginary meridians in the body to keep the body nourished. The meridians correspond to specific human organs: kidneys, liver, spleen, heart, lungs, pericardium, bladder, gall bladder, stomach, small and large intestines, and the triple burner (body temperature regulator). It is believed that blocked meridians cause illness or pain. When the channels are open, life energy flows smoothly and you experience optimal health

To use acupressure, you place your thumbs or index finger on certain "points" along the body's meridians, using firm but gentle pressure. (There are about 12,000 acu-points.) Hold this pressure for several seconds, and then move to another point. Many of the body's acu-points are near nerves. When the nerves are stimulated, it causes a dull ache or pressure in the muscle. This, in turn, triggers a message to the central nervous system and causes the release of endorphins and monoamines, the chemicals that block pain signals in the spinal cord and the brain. Acupressure is also thought to trigger the release of serotonin, a brain chemical that makes you feel calm and serene. After experiencing acupressure, you may experience less muscle tension, increased blood circulation, and a reduced amount of pain.

Today acupressure is used to relieve everyday aches, pains, and stress, as well as specific conditions like sinus pressure, leg cramps, tension headaches, temporomandibular joint disorder (TMJ), back and neck pain, and carpal tunnel syndrome.

Acupuncture Releases Serotonin and Norepinephrine

My patient Susan turned to alternative therapies for migraine relief when her prescribed medications made her feel drowsy and inattentive. After trying everything from shots to nasal sprays to strong narcotics, this forty-two-year-old registered nurse and mother finally got long-term relief with regular acupuncture treatments.

Acupuncture is the insertion of one or more dry needles into the skin and underlying tissues at specific acupuncture points. When the needles are gently twisted or stimulated, a measurable release of endorphins may go into the bloodstream, energy blocks are removed, and the flow of energy along the meridians is restored. Various endorphins block incoming pain information through the release of serotonin and norepinephrine. Some researchers suggest that peripheral nerve stimulation can modify functional responses within the brain. In this way, the patient's pain tolerance is increased so that one acupuncture treatment in some patients may help alleviate chronic pain for weeks. Studies have shown that acupuncture may alter brain chemistry by changing the release of neurotransmitters that stimulate or inhibit nerve impulses in the brain that relay information about external stimuli and sensations (such as pain) in a good way.

Another way of stimulating the acupuncture points once the needle is in place is by hooking up small wires connected to very slight electrical currents. This is known as electro-acupuncture. Heat (moxibustion) and massage (acupressure) can be used during this process. Laser acupuncture is yet another off-shoot of this alternative therapy and is particularly well-suited for the treatment of carpal tunnel syndrome. While it uses the same points, there are no needles involved.

In a report published in the June 2001 issue of the *British Medical Journal*, researchers concluded that acupuncture was an effective treatment for chronic neck pain. In the study, about 200 patients were given either acupuncture treatments, massage therapy, or a sham laser acupuncture for thirty minutes, five times a week for three weeks. During follow-up examinations, more than half of those treated with acupuncture reported a more than 50 percent improvement in pain related to motion. These individuals even reported relief from pain immediately after one acupuncture treatment, and one week after the treatments were completed.

According to a National Institutes of Health consensus panel in November 1997, acupuncture may be useful by itself or combined with conventional therapies to treat addiction, headaches, menstrual cramps, tennis elbow, fibromyalgia, myofascial pain, osteoarthritis, lower back pain, carpal tunnel syndrome, and asthma; and to assist in stroke rehabilitation.

If you want to try acupuncture for chronic pain relief, make sure you get a licensed acupuncturist who uses only disposable needles. Acupuncture tends to be operator-dependent, therefore choose a practitioner who has a lot of experience. In addition, there are multiple styles, depending on where the practitioner studied. For instance, Chinese acupuncture depends on larger bore needles and the practitioner may be more aggressive with moving them. Japanese acupuncture uses thinner bore needles with a relatively gentle approach. Find the style that suits your needs.

Acupuncture has very few contraindications, and the side effects are small. At this time, in the United States there are more than 6,500 certified and licensed practitioners and more than 3,000 of these are conventional medical doctors. For recommendations, you can contact the American Academy of Medical Acupuncture (AAMA). This organization, founded in 1987, restricts membership to those who have more than 220 hours of formal training and are medical doctors (M.D.s) and doctors of osteopathy (D.O.s). Check out their Web site at www.medicalacupuncture.org.

Shiatsu

Shiatsu is another healing touch therapy that works similarly to acupressure and acupuncture. This ancient Japanese therapy has been found to ease headaches, back and neck pain, and muscle pain.

Unlike acupressure and acupuncture, the shiatsu practitioner works with your deep breathing, and rhythmically applies gentle to deep pressure to specific points (called "tsubos") on the body's meridians. This pressure may be applied with palms, fingers, elbows, knees and feet, but most practitioners work with their thumbs held side by side or, for more concentrated pressure, on top of one another.

Ayurvedic Massage

Ayurvedic massage is yet another ancient therapy that is useful for alleviating chronic pain and increasing relaxation. This ancient Indian remedy is said to unblock invisible "marma" points in the body through which energy flows. When this energy is freed, your body will heal itself.

Today Abhayanga massage (oil massage) is offered at many spas throughout the world. Using special herbal oil chosen for your particular *dosha* (metabolic type), two therapists massage you at the same time. This intense touch therapy is followed by an energetic rubdown with a coarse towel.

Other Common Touch Therapies

Reflexology

Reflexology works along the same principle as acupressure and shiatsu. This ancient healing art is based on the theory that reflex zones on the feet correspond with specific zones or organs in the body. By massaging or manipulating the zones on the feet with your thumb, fingers, or hands, you can influence healing in the body. For instance, according to reflexology theory, massaging the outer side of the foot may ease any ailment or pain you feel in your back. Alternatively, massaging the big toe may ease a chronic headache. The following chart shows how reflexology corresponds to different body zones.

Reflex Point	Corresponding Body Zone
Metatarsal (balls of the feet)	Chest, lung, and shoulder area
Toes	Head and neck

Upper arch	Diaphragm, upper abdominal organs
Lower arch	Pelvic and lower abdominal organs
Heel	Pelvic and sciatic nerve
Outer foot	Arm, shoulder, hip, leg, knee, and lower back
Inner foot	Spine
Ankle area	Reproductive organs and pelvic region

Reiké

Reiké is a technique practiced by experienced practitioners known as reike masters who "funnel their energy through their hands" and attempt to ease pain by applying their minds to painful areas.

Therapeutic Touch

In this technique there is generally no actual touching, but the experienced therapeutic touch practitioner attempts to use their hands near and around the body to restore normal "energy flow patterns."

Chiropractic

Chiropractic care is a very common alternative therapy for chronic pain and may be helpful for treating back pain, chronic cervicogenic or musculoskeletal headaches, neck pain, and pain from musculoskeletal injuries. This therapy may be effective for fibromyalgia, as it helps improve pain levels and increase cervical and lumbar ranges of motion.

As the largest alternative medical profession, chiropractic is based on the principle that the body is a self-healing organism. To reduce pain and increase healing, the doctor of chiropractic uses spinal adjustments with the goal of increasing the mobility between spinal vertebrae, which have become restricted, locked, or slightly out of proper position. Chiropractors do this by using hand adjustments with gentle pressure or stretching, multiple gentle movements of one area or specific high-velocity thrusts. Adjustments are said to help return the bones to a more normal position or motion, helping to relieve pain and reduce ill health.

If you try chiropractic, you might have quick relief immediately after manipulation or it may take weeks to receive a benefit. In some situations, it may not work at all. Still, whether or not you find relief from chiropractic manipulation, it is important to continue with the rest of the complete holistic program, including your doctor's pre-scribed medications, if needed.

Does Bodywork Really Work?

Bodywork is the umbrella term that describes the hands-on tech-nique of massage, touch, and movement used to align the spine, muscles, and joints to promote the flow of energy. This alternative therapy promotes relaxation, especially with the musculoskeletal system, enhances the circulation of blood and lymph, and relieves muscle tension.

Bodywork includes more than 150 varieties of body manipula-tion therapies used for relaxation and pain relief. Of these, massage therapy, the scientific manipulation of the body's soft tissues to normalize those tissues, is perhaps the most popular—and with reason. A massage can make you feel incredibly relaxed, boost pain-relieving endorphins, and distract you from any chronic pain or negative feelings. With massage, the therapist applies manual techniques to the muscles, fascia, tendons, and ligaments with the goal of healing the body. Some of the methods used include rub-bing, kneading, tapping, manipulating, holding, friction pressure, taping, and vibrating.

If you wish to use massage therapy, make sure you use a licensed therapist, if possible. Go to the American Massage Therapy Associ-ation's Web site at www.amtamassage.org or call them at 888-843-2682 for more information.

Types of Massage

Here are a few popular types of massage to ease pain:

Swedish massage is a type of hands-on touch in which the practi-tioner uses a system of long strokes, kneading, and friction tech-niques to massage the more superficial layers of the muscles. Swedish massage is combined with active and passive movements of the joints, and oil is usually used, which facilitates the stroking and kneading of the body, thereby stimulating metabolism and circula-tion. The therapist applies pressure and rubs the muscles in the same direction as the flow of blood returning to the heart.

The many benefits of Swedish massage include increased relaxation, greater mobility of joints, decreased muscle tightness, and improved circulation. No matter what type of pain you have, this soothing massage will help you relax—and that can help anyone sleep better and enjoy improved mood.

Deep tissue massage may be helpful for women with fibromyalgia, especially because the therapist uses greater pressure than Swedish massage and targets the deep layers of muscle. Using a series of slow strokes and direct pressure, the therapist will strive to release chronic patterns of muscular tension. Sometimes the therapists use their elbows or thumbs to push hard into the deepest grain of the muscle in order to reduce tension.

Neuromuscular massage combines the basic principles of ancient Asian therapies, such as acupressure and shiatsu, along with specific hands-on deep tissue therapy to help reduce chronic muscle or myofascial (soft-tissue) pain.

Body Education

There are some excellent types of bodywork that can help you relearn good posture and get your body in balance, to take pressure off painful joints and muscles. This type of "body education" may help those who have repetitive stress injuries, as you relearn how to sit correctly and move your body during daily activities. Bodywork can be beneficial for women who suffer with chronic hip, knee, back, or neck pain. There are many types of bodywork, but here are a few types that may be helpful for relief of chronic pain:

Rolfing is a holistic system of massage and manipulation of the body's myofascial system that is said to dramatically alter a person's posture and structure. Rolfing is said to ease chronic pain and improve performance of athletes, dancers, actors, and others who depend on physical strength and proper movements for their life's work.

Aston-Patterning, an offshoot of Rolfing's deep-tissue massage, focuses on an ergonomically sound workplace and home environment. This type of body education helps you to be aware of how you stand, walk, sit, bend, reach, and lift. The practitioner will give the massage and then, according to your physical measurements, coach you in how to relearn ways of moving.

The Trager Approach is targeted at those with chronic pain. Using a series of gentle, nonintrusive movements, the practitioner will jiggle, rock, and vibrate your limbs and musculature, while you are in a reclining position, to increase mobility and deep relaxation. You'll have homework with Trager, to help reinforce the classroom lessons.

The Felderkrais Method was developed by Moshe Feldenkrais, a Polish-born physicist who had to relearn how to walk after suffering a crippling knee injury. Feldenkrais Method is based on the theory that the brain and nervous system choose the most "energy-efficient" way of moving. Sometimes bad habits cause us to move incorrectly and can result in unnecessary pain. During sessions, the therapist works with you to help you increase flexibility and "re-teach" your brain and body how to work together so you'll feel the difference between the old patterns and the new, more efficient ones.

The Alexander Technique is a method of analyzing the way you move your body, then enabling you to change old patterns that may be causing pain and distress. For instance, if you tend to slump at your desk, the teacher would help you recognize this bad habit and help you learn and practice healthy posture. You will also learn how to stand, walk, lift, and bend without stressing your body.

As you have read, the choices for mind/body therapies to help reduce stress and anxiety and control pain are numerous. Review the therapies in this step and select one or two that you feel might benefit your situation. Use these therapies daily, following the instructions, until you are able to move into a relaxed mode at will—whether sitting in a line of rush hour traffic, waiting for a doctor's appointment, or leading a meeting at work. If the mind/body therapy is right for you, you should notice improvement quickly with reduced stress symptoms, increased healing sleep, and hopefully, less pain. Continue to schedule time daily to do the exercises for optimal benefit.

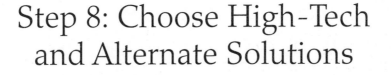

CHAPTER SIXTEEN

Step 8: Choose High-Tech and Alternate Solutions

Most women with chronic pain are able to control their pain using the holistic program of medications, diet, exercise, and natural therapies. Still, there are times when more "high-tech" solutions are necessary. For instance, you may benefit from an electronic gadget that helps to increase blood flow to the painful site or one that breaks the cycle of pain. Surgery may be necessary to correct an anatomical problem. For example, if you have severe osteoarthritis of the knee, knee replacement surgery may give you back your active life. If you suffer with painful menstrual cramps from endometriosis or fibroid tumors, surgical procedures to correct these problems may enable you to live pain-free and enjoy an improved quality of life.

Whether or not you need a surgical procedure is between you and your doctor. In this last step in my program, I will introduce you to some high-tech measures that may reduce your pain, as well as guide you through a reasonable process for evaluating a surgeon and facility, if a surgical procedure is necessary.

To decide if you are a good candidate for surgery, you must consider the level of pain you feel and how it has affected your quality of life. If your pain is constant and incapacitating, and if activity or exercise is limited even with nonoperative treatment, surgery may be a consideration.

A good test method to help you determine if a high-tech treatment is necessary is to use a calendar to chart the days when your pain either is immobilizing or prevents you from doing your daily tasks and activities. Using the following calendar, circle those days when the pain is immobilizing or incapacitating. Look back over this calendar in three weeks. If more days are circled than not, and if the pain is not starting to diminish, you should talk to your doctor to see if a high-tech or surgical procedure may help you.

PAIN CALENDAR						
1	2	3	4	5	6	7
8	9	10	11	12	13	14
15	16	17	18	19	20	21

High-Tech Pain Busters

I use these various high-tech gadgets with my patients to help ease many types of chronic back, knee, shoulder, neck, and muscle pain, as well as pain from work-related injuries, such as carpal tunnel syndrome. These pain busters may be used alone or in combination with other treatments.

Injections

Various types of injections may occasionally be useful for certain painful conditions (e.g. peripheral nerve blocks, sympathetic nerve blocks, bursal injections, joint injections).

Trigger Point Injections (TPI).   Trigger point injections are sometimes given for neck pain, headaches, and low back pain to treat muscle spasm and other soft tissue problems. These injections of medications, such as a local anesthetic or cortisone derivative, are given directly into the painful site to alleviate pain and inflammation.

Epidural Injections.   Other injections around the spine (epidural injections of a cortisone derivative and anesthetic) can be used in some cases for constant, severe pain. These injections may give weeks of relief for women who suffer with chronic back pain, especially with lower extremity pain and other related back or hip pain.

Facet Joint Injection.   This type of injection (usually a long-lasting steroid) helps to ease certain types of low back pain. It goes right into the facet joints, which are located in the back and neck at each vertebral level.

Sacroiliac Joint Injection. This is an injection of cortisone (a steroid) in the sacroiliac joints, located in the back where the lumbosacral spine joins the pelvis. This injection helps to relieve some types of pain in the low back, buttocks, abdomen, groin, and legs.

Botulinum Toxin. Botulinum toxin functions as a therapeutic muscle-relaxing agent when it's injected into the muscle to help relieve pain. Derived from the bacterium *Clostridium botulinum*, botulinum toxin works at motor nerve endings (nerves that lead to muscles). Pain relief may be from a blocking action on the release of neurotransmitters. Botulinum toxin appears to produce prolonged muscle relaxation and can be targeted to the particular muscle group associated with the pain. In some patients with migraine and tension headaches, botulinum toxin injections have led to significantly more headache-free days and a decline in pain intensity. Botulinum toxin is available as two types: Botulinum toxin serotype A (Botox) and Botulinum toxin serotype B (Myobloc).

Longer Term Narcotic Injection. In some unusual cases of chronic pain, surgical-type procedures can be used to insert a catheter for long-term use of narcotics or other drugs for pain control. A device called a port is installed, usually on the abdomen, which allows injections of medication as often as needed. The pump installed through surgery can also allow medication (such as morphine) to be delivered continuously for additional pain relief. Rarely, continuous infusions of narcotics, such as morphine and/or other medications can be infused into the spine.

Ultrasound

Ultrasound uses sound waves delivered at a frequency above the human range of hearing that are applied to the muscles, tendons, and other soft tissues of the back. This may help increase relaxation, decrease inflammation, and improve pain of tender points. Ultrasound is more commonly used for acute back pain and other similar situations than for chronic pain. However, if you try it and it gives relief, ultrasound can be done by a physical therapist.

Galvanic Ultrasound. This noninvasive therapy uses high-frequency sound waves combined with high-voltage pulsed galvanic stimulation to alleviate pain and increase blood flow at injured sites on the body.

Electronic Stimulation

Transcutaneous Electrical Nerve Stimulation (TENS).   With TENS, electrical impulses are sent to certain nerves that block the messages of pain being sent by other nerves from the painful area. These impulses might also cause the body to release endorphins, which are natural pain relievers produced by the body. Different settings can be tried and one may work better than others.

With TENS, you wear a stimulator and battery, usually on a belt. Electrical wires from the stimulator attach to electrodes held by adhesive (usually a patch) on the skin. The electrodes are placed in the area of pain but may need to be tried at different locations to get the best relief.

The TENS unit can be used throughout most of the day (for example, one hour on, one hour off) or only as needed for the pain. Usually there will be a trial of about one month to see the effect on pain.

Percutaneous Electrical Nerve Stimulation (PENS).   PENS therapy uses acupuncturelike needle probes in the soft tissues to stimulate peripheral sensory nerves. PENS may be preferred over TENS in that it delivers the electrical stimulus in closer proximity to the nerve endings located in the soft tissue. This form of analgesic therapy may be useful for those with migraine headache and chronic lower back pain.

Electro-acupuncture.   Electro-acupuncture uses stimulation of specific trigger points on the body with small electrical impulses (milliamp/microamp) through acupuncture needles or with electrostim hand-held cutaneous probes. It is different from TENS because it uses a lower voltage cutaneous stimulation and is used to treat back and shoulder pain, headache, fibromyalgia, muscle pain, and arthritis pain, among others.

Intradiscal ElectroThermal Treatment.   When chronic back pain results from nerve growth into the cracks of a torn disc in the lumbar spine (e.g. discogenic pain), your doctor may believe that fusion surgery is the only way to resolve this problem. In this type of surgery, the degenerated disc is removed and the vertebrae are fused together in a single piece. However, findings published in the May 2002 issue of the journal *Spine* may help you avoid surgery altogether. In the study, researchers found that Intradiscal Electro Thermal Treatment (IDET) helps shrink and contract the collagen protein surrounding the disc and virtually stimulates the disc to heal itself. With IDET, a catheter with an attached heating element is passed through a thin needle into the degenerated disc. Using heat, the surgeon seals the cracks and cauterizes the nerves that send pain messages to the brain, resulting in less pain and a greater quality of life. Although the exact mechanisms of pain relief are uncertain and this therapy is too new to advocate it as being a proven effective therapy, it appears that under certain circumstances IDET may provide some benefit when it is used in conjunction with a specific post-IDET therapy program.

Neuromodulation. In some conditions, implanted peripheral nerve stimulators or spinal cord stimulators may be helpful for severe intractable pain.

Your Surgical Assessment

If your doctor claims surgery is the only way for you to live pain-free, then do some homework ahead of time to make sure you have the most qualified surgeon and a reputable facility. Surgery is just the beginning of your process to resolve pain. There's still a lot of work ahead as you prepare for the procedure and follow the rehabilitation plan after surgery. In some cases, serious risks are involved such as bleeding, blood clots, or even an adverse result from the surgery. Make sure you understand this ahead of time and are willing to accept any risks involved.

To keep the complications or risks of surgery low, consult with your primary-care physician or internist to make sure other considerations—such as heart problems, lung disease, a chronic illness such as diabetes, or your age—do not put you at high risk for surgery. Let your doctor guide you as you make the safest choice.

Moreover, always get a second opinion. Speaking with another doctor about your pain situation may give you new insight in how to resolve it. Different doctors have varying opinions regarding surgery, and hearing both sides will help you make an educated decision.

Ask for Referrals and Interview Surgeons

Ask your doctor for the names of well-skilled surgeons, as well as for the names of highly regarded hospitals and outpatient surgical facilities. In some cases, travel may be involved. Check with your health care provider to see if the professionals and services needed are covered under your plan.

Medicine is changing dramatically. In years past we relied on our doctors to provide medical care and keep us well. However, the traditional, autocratic role of doctors is now challenged by millions of people as they seek to make informed choices regarding their bodies and necessary health care. While you may feel uncomfortable interviewing a surgeon and asking pertinent, even personal, questions regarding his or her knowledge and experience, you must do it to find a professional with whom you can trust your life.

Do Your Homework

Over the telephone, you can find out if the recommended surgeons are board-certified, which means that the doctors have passed a standard exam given by the governing board in their specialties, and where the doctors attended medical school. Your local medical society will provide this information. Sometimes it is a plus if the doctor is involved in any academic pursuits, such as teaching, writing, or research, as this surgeon may be more up-to-date in the latest developments in his or her field. Find out where the doctor has hospital privileges and where these hospitals are located. Some doctors may not admit patients to certain hospitals, an important consideration, especially if you have a chronic health problem. You should also consider how many surgeries this physician has done for your particular problem. For example, if you are having back surgery to repair a ruptured disc, twenty-five to thirty previous surgeries should be a minimum requirement.

Plan a Consultation

Once you have narrowed down your search, plan an initial consultation with the surgeon, during which you can get to know each other. This consultation will include a detailed interview and physical examination. To make certain the surgeon fully understands your problem and your overall health, bring the following with you:

- Copies of any X rays, CT scans, or MRI scans
- All lab results
- Your medical files
- A comprehensive list of any medications you are taking (or have recently taken)

- A list of any natural dietary supplements, including herbs, you are taking (or have recently taken)
- A list of any known allergies (including latex allergy or allergy to medications)

Talk openly about your needs, and ask the surgeon what the chances are for pain relief. Be specific with questions about exercise and increasing activity. If you want to be able to play golf or tennis, ask whether it will be possible after surgery. If you are contemplating getting pregnant, be upfront and ask if this will be possible after surgery. If you cannot do your job, which entails bending and lifting, ask if surgery will help you at work. Good patient-physician communication is important for receiving the highest quality of care and the comfort needed during anxious moments before surgery. Many patients find it helpful to write down their questions ahead of time, so they are less apt to forget these at the time of consultation.

During the examination, find out about the preferred method of surgery. Is the surgeon current in using the latest methods? Will the surgeon allow patient-controlled analgesia (PCA), which means you control the amount of pain medication used after surgery? Ask if the surgeon will perform all of the surgery. If not, how much will be done by the surgeon's assistant, physician's assistant, or hospital resident? Also, find out if this doctor will be on call after surgery, or if another doctor will see you.

Choose an Accredited Hospital

Depending on the type of surgery you require, the procedure may be done in your surgeon's office or at an outpatient facility, into which you will be admitted for surgery, then leave the same day. Or you may be admitted to a hospital for inpatient surgery. If your surgery is elective and if you have time, go to this chosen facility or hospital and assess the cleanliness. Ask around to find out its reputation, and whether it is accredited by the Joint Commission on Accreditation of Healthcare Organization (JCAHO). This commission evaluates and accredits more than fifteen thousand health care organizations across the United States, including hospitals and ambulatory health care centers.

Check Out the Costs

Not only is surgery stressful, it's also outrageously expensive. That's why doing your homework could save you a great deal of stress when the bills start to come in. Get in writing at least an estimate of the cost of the surgery, including hospital stay and follow-up therapy, and check with your insurance company to see how much of the surgery will be covered by your plan. Unforeseen expenses can create a considerable financial burden, so it's best to know what you'll have to pay ahead of time.

Meet the Anesthesiologist

If your surgery is to be immediate, you may not have the chance to talk at length with your anesthesiologist. This doctor specializes in the elimination of pain and sensation for patients undergoing surgery, and maintains your life while the normal triggers for breathing are anesthetized. However, if you are planning for surgery, it is standard to meet with this person during the preoperative exam. Whether you meet your anesthesiologist a week ahead or only five minutes before surgery, make sure he or she knows the following:

- Other health problems you may have (lung disease, heart problems, chronic illness)
- Problems with anesthesia or intubation in the past
- Your desire to be awake (or not) during surgery
- Allergies
- Problems such as malignant hyperthermia or latex allergy
- Medications you are taking, including blood thinners, herbs, and dietary supplements

Local or General Anesthesia?

Anesthesia is used during surgery so you will feel no pain or discomfort. Three types of anesthesia are generally used: local, regional, and general. Each type usually attempts to block the process through which pain signals are sent from the affected nerves to the spinal cord and to the brain.

Many anesthesiologists use local anesthetics and regional blocks during surgery; this choice may help reduce the chances of various complications in certain patients. These types of anesthesia may be of particular benefit to those with heart or lung problems, but not necessarily; discuss your options with your anesthesiologist.

A local anesthetic (nerve block) will block nerve sensations in a specific area of the body. A spinal or epidural block involves numbing with an anesthetic such as lidocaine. It may involve putting a catheter into the epidural space in the spinal column. This catheter will enable the doctor to anesthetize a larger portion of the body and to continue injecting local anesthetic or administer continuous infusion for a long period of time—even into the post-operative period. The epidural infusion into the post-operative period (after surgery) may enable you to participate more in pain control, physical therapy, and rehabilitation in efforts to speed recovery.

General anesthesia, which produces an unconscious state, affects your entire system and takes time to wear off. Very rarely it can have dangerous side effects for some, but if properly done, it is extremely safe to use.

Types of Surgery

If your final option for pain relief is surgery, it's important to know that each type of surgery has a specific advantage, depending on the severity and location of the problem and such factors as your age or other chronic illnesses.

Open surgery, using a scalpel, may require a few days to a week in the hospital, general anesthesia, and three weeks to three months of recovery time, including physical therapy.

Minimally invasive surgery is a technique that does not require a large incision. This allows recovery time to be faster, and you may only stay in the hospital or facility for a few hours as an outpatient. Some types of minimally invasive surgery include the following:

- Laparoscopy: Uses a tube with a light and a camera lens at the end (laparoscope) to look at internal organs, check for abnormalities, or perform surgical procedures.
- Endoscopy: Uses a small flexible tube with a light and a camera lens at the end (endoscope) to examine the inside of the digestive tract.
- Arthroscopy: Uses an endoscope to examine the interior of a joint and make surgical corrections, if necessary.

- Cystoscopy: Uses an endoscope to examine the inside of the urethra and bladder cavity to check for abnormalities.
- Gastroscopy: Uses an endoscope to examine the lining of the stomach.
- Sigmoidoscopy: Uses endoscope to examine the rectum and sigmoid colon.
- Colonoscopy: Uses an colonoscope to examine the entire large intestine, from the lowest part, the rectum, all the way up through the colon to the lower end of the small intestine.
- Laser surgery: Directs a powerful beam of light to specific parts of the body without making a large incision. The laser heat seals blood vessels so bleeding is minimal, and the recovery time for laser surgery is generally less than open surgery.

However, no matter how minimally invasive the procedure appears, you will still be expected to follow the doctor's orders on rehabilitation and physical therapy. You may still need to take the prescribed medications to keep swelling down and halt pain. Be sure to let your doctor guide you as you choose the type of surgery that is best to help you end pain and regain an active life.

Consider a Comprehensive Pain Clinic

If you've exhausted all of the pain-relieving methods and are still suffering with chronic pain, you may want to seek support from a comprehensive pain program. Most pain clinics use a multifaceted approach to treatment, which includes a combination of medical and physical therapies, as well as psychological approaches to control pain.

At a comprehensive pain clinic, you may receive an evaluation by a variety of healthcare professionals, possibly including a neurologist, rheumatologist, anesthesiologist, physical medicine specialist, orthopedist, gynecologist, and psychologist, among others. These doctors will work in consultation with each other to devise the best plan to relieve your pain. For instance, using a combination of medications, exercise, physical therapy, relaxation treatments, acupuncture, and psychotherapy, you may finally get optimal pain relief.

By the time most women decide to use a pain clinic, they are often desperate for help. In some cases, women suffer with depression from the chronic pain or might have a history of drug abuse because of the addictive nature of some effective pain-relieving drugs. Experts at pain clinics are aware of the emotional and medical complications that stem from chronic pain. These men and women will use every conventional and alternative avenue to provide you with excellent care with the goal of returning to a normal, active life.

I wish you the best of luck on your journey.

References

Aaron, L.A., Burke, M.M., Buchwald, D. Overlapping conditions among patients with chronic fatigue syndrome, fibromyalgia, and temporomandibular disorder. *Archives of Internal Medicine* 2000; 160:221.

ACOG Practice Bulletin Number 11. *Medical Management of Endometriosis.* December 1999.

Adler, G.K., Kinsley, B.T., Hurwitz, S., et al. Reduced hypothalamic-pituitary and sympathoadrenal responses to hypoglycemia in women with fibromyalgia syndrome. *American Journal of Medicine* 1999; 106:534.

Arnold, M., et al. A randomized, placebo-controlled, double-blind, flexible-dose study of fluoxetine in the treatment of women with fibromyalgia. *American Journal of Medicine* 2002 Feb 15;112(3):191–7.

Atroshi, I., Gummesson, C., Johnsson, R., Ornstein, E. Prevalence of carpal tunnel syndrome in a general population. *Journal of the American Medical Association* 1999; 282:153.

Bandt, M.D. Vitamin E uncouples joint destruction and clinical inflammation in a transgenic mouse model of rheumatoid arthritis. *Arthritis and Rheumatism* 2002 Feb;46(2):522–32.

Barbour C. Use of complementary and alternative treatments by individuals with fibromyalgia syndrome. *Journal of the American Academy of Nurse Practitioners* 2000 Aug;12(8):311–6.

Barkhuizen A. Pharmacologic Treatment of Fibromyalgia. *Current Pain and Headache Reports* 2001 Aug;5(4):351–8.

Barnard, N.D., Scialli, A.R., Hurlock, D., Bertron, P. Diet and sex-hormone binding globulin, dysmenorrhea, and premenstrual symptoms. *Obstetrics and Gynecology* 2000; 95:245.

Belch, J.J., et al. Evening primrose oil and borage oil in rheumatologic conditions. *American Journal of Clinical Nutrition* 2000 Jan;71(1 Suppl):352S-6S.

Bennett, R.M. Emerging concepts in the neurobiology of chronic pain: Evidence of abnormal sensory processing in fibromyalgia. *Mayo Clinic Proceedings* 1999; 74:385.

Benson, H., et al. Relaxation Response: Bridge Between Psychiatry and Medicine. *Medical Clinics of North America (1977)* 61:929–938.

Buskila D. Fibromyalgia, chronic fatigue syndrome, and myofascial pain syndrome. *Current Opinions in Rheumatology* 2000;12:113–123.

Byrne, C., Connolly, J.L., Colditz, G.A., Schnitt, S.J. Biopsy confirmed benign breast disease, postmenopausal use of exogenous female hormones, and breast carcinoma risk. *Cancer* 2000; 89:2046.

Capobianco, D.J., Cheshire, W.P., Campbell, J.K. An overview of the diagnosis and pharmacologic treatment of migraine. *Mayo Clinic Proceedings* 1996; 71:1055.

Carette, S., Leclaire, R., Marcoux, E.S., et al. Epidural corticosteroid injections for sciatica due to herniated nucleus pulposus. *New England Journal of Medicine* 1997; 336:1634.

Castleman, M. The Healing Herbs. *The Ultimate Guide to the Curative Power of Nature's Medicines.* (New York: Bantam Books 1995) p.27.

Cherkin, D.C., Deyo, R.A., Battie, M. A comparison of physical therapy, chiropractic manipulation, and provision of an educational booklet for the treatment of patients with low back pain. *New England Journal of Medicine* 1998; 339:1021.

Cherkin, D.C., Eisenberg, D., Sherman, K.J., et al. Randomized trial comparing traditional Chinese medical acupuncture, therapeutic massage, and self-care education for chronic low back pain. *Archives of Internal Medicine* 2001; 161:1081.

Cho, Z.H., et al. New findings of the correlation between acupoints and corresponding brain cortices using functional MRI. *Proceedings of the National Academy of Sciences of the United States of America*, 1998 Mar 3, 95(5):2670–3.

Chugani, D.C., et al. Increased brain serotonin synthesis in migraine. *Neurology* 1999; 53:1473.

Crofford, Leslie J., and Clauw, Daniel J. Fibromyalgia: Where are we a decade after the American College of Rheumatology classification criteria were developed? *Arthritis and Rheumatism* 2002 Volume 46, Issue 5, 1136–1138.

Cutler, N., et al. Oral sumatriptan for the acute treatment of migraine: evaluation of three dosage strengths. *Neurology* 1995; 45:S5.

Deyo, R.A., et al. A controlled trial of transcutaneous electrical nerve stimulation (TENS) and exercise for chronic low back pain. *New England Journal of Medicine* 1990; 322:1627.

Drukker, B.H. Fibrocystic change of the breast. *Clinical Obstetrics and Gynecology* 1994; 37:903.

Dunn, K.S., et al. The Prevalence of Prayer as a Spiritual Self-care Modality in Elders. *Journal of Holistic Nursing* (December 2000) 18(4):337–51.

Eisenberg, D.M. Advising patients who seek alternative medical therapies. *Annals of Internal Medicine* 1997; 127:61.

Ferraccioli, G., et al. EMG-biofeedback training in fibromyalgia syndrome. *Journal of Rheumatology* 1987; 14:820.

Ferry, S., et al. Carpal tunnel syndrome: a nested case-control study of risk factors in women. *American Journal of Epidemiology* 2000; 151:566.

Foster, L., et al. Botulinum toxin A and chronic low back pain: a randomized, double-blind study. *Neurology* 2001; 56:1290.

Garfinkel, M.S., Schumacher, H.R., Husain, A., et al. Evaluation of a yoga based regimen for treatment of osteoarthritis of the hands. *Journal of Rheumatology* 1994; 21:2341.

Hadhazy, V.A., Ezzo, J., Creamer, P., Berman, B.M. Mind-body therapies for the treatment of fibromyalgia. A systematic review. *Journal of Rheumatology* 2000; 27:2911.

Haqqi, Tarig M., et al. Prevention of collagen-induced arthritis in mice by a polyphenolic fraction from green tea. *Proceedings of the National Academy of Science* 1999 Vol. 96, Issue 8, 4524–4529.

Hanninen, Kaartinen K., et al. Antioxidants in vegan diet and rheumatic disorders. *Toxicology* 2000 Nov 30;155(1–3):45–53.

Hansen, C.J., et al. Exercise Duration and Mood State: How Much Is Enough to Feel Better? *Health Psychology 2001* Jul;20(4):267–75.

Hardy, M., et al. Replacement of Drug Therapy for Insomnia by Ambient Odor. *Lancet* (1995) 346:701.

Hathcock, J.N. Does high intake of vitamin A pose a risk for osteoporotic fracture? *Journal of the American Medical Association.* 2002 Mar 20;287(11):1396–7.

Holroyd, Kenneth, et al. Management of Chronic Tension-Type Headache With Tricyclic Antidepressant Medication, Stress Management Therapy, and Their Combination: A Randomized Controlled Trial. *Journal of the American Medical Association* 2001;285:2208–2215.

Ironson, G., et al. Massage Therapy is Associated with Enhancement of the Immune System's Cytotoxic Capacity. *International Journal of Neuroscience.* (February 1996) 84(1–4):205–17.

Jonas, W.B. The effect of niacinamide on osteoarthritis: a pilot study. *Inflammatory Research* 1996 Jul;45(7):330–4.

Kent, D.L., Haynor, D.R., Longstreth, W.T. Jr., et al. The clinical efficacy of magnetic resonance imaging in neuroimaging. *Annals of Internal Medicine* 1994; 120:856.

Keville, Kathi, and Green, Mindy. *Aromatherapy: A Complete Guide to the Healing Art.* (Santa Cruz, California: Crossing Press, 1995).

Korszun, A., Sackett-Lundeen, L., Papadopoulos, E., et al. Melatonin levels in women with fibromyalgia and chronic fatigue syndrome. *Journal of Rheumatology* 1999; 26:2675.

Kremer, J.M. n-3 fatty acid supplements in rheumatoid arthritis. *American Journal of Clinical Nutrition* 2000 Jan;71(1 Suppl):349S-51S.

Lane, A.M., et al. The effects of exercise on mood changes: the moderating effect of depressed mood. *Journal of Sports Medicine and Physical Fitness* 2001 Dec;41(4):539–45.

Pei, J. and Sun, L., et al. The effect of electro-acupuncture on motor function recovery in patients with acute cerebral infarction: a randomly controlled trial. *Journal of Traditional Chinese Medicine* 2001 Dec;21(4):270–2.

Perez-Ruiz, F., Calabozo, M., Alonso-Ruiz, A., et al. High prevalence of undetected carpal tunnel syndrome in patients with fibromyalgia syndrome. *Journal of Rheumatology* 1995; 22:501.

Proctor, M.L., Roberts, H., Farquhar, C.M. Combined oral contraceptive pill (OCP) as treatment for primary dysmenorrhoea (Cochrane Review). *Cochrane Database of Systematic Reviews* 2001; 4:CD002120.

Ramalanjaona, Georges. Magnesium in the Treatment of Fibromyalgia. *Alternative Medicine Alert* March 2002.

Ray, U.S., et al. Effect of Yogic Exercises on Physical and Mental Health of Young Fellowship Course Trainees. *Indian Journal of Physiology and Pharmacology* 2001 Jan;45(1):37–53.

Reid, I.R., et al. Intravenous Zoledronic Acid in Postmenopausal Women with Low Bone Mineral Density. *New England Journal of Medicine* 2002; 346:653–661.

Reginster, J-Y., Deroisy, R., Paul, I., et al. Glucosamine sulfate significantly reduces progression of knee osteoarthritis over 3 years: A large, randomized, placebo-controlled, double-blind, prospective trial. *Arthritis and Rheumatology* 1999; 42:S400.

Roizenblatt, S., et al. Alpha sleep characteristics in fibromyalgia. *Arthritis and Rheumatism* 2001;44:222–230.

Rooks, D.S., et al. The effects of progressive strength training and aerobic exercise on muscle strength and cardiovascular fitness in women with fibromyalgia: a pilot study. *Arthritis and Rheumatism* 2002 Feb; 47(1):22–8.

Russell, I.J., Orr, M.D., Littman, B., et al. Elevated cerebrospinal fluid levels of substance P in patients with the fibromyalgia syndrome. *Arthritis and Rheumatism* 1994; 37:1593.

Schmidt, W.D., et al. Effects of long versus short bout exercise on fitness and weight loss in overweight females. *Journal of the American College of Nutrition* 2001 Oct;20(5):494–501.

Schulman, E.A., Cady, R.K., Henry, D., et al. Effectiveness of sumatriptan in reducing productivity loss due to migraine: Results of a randomized, double-blind, placebo-controlled clinical trial. *Mayo Clinic Proceedings* 2000; 75:782.

Sherman, J.J., et al. Nonpharmacologic Approaches to the Management of Myofascial Temporomandibular Disorders. *Current Pain and Headache Report* (October 2001) 5(5):421–31.

Smetana, G.W. The diagnostic value of historical features in primary headache syndromes: a comprehensive review. *Archives of Internal Medicine* 2000; 160:2729.

Smith, J.D., et al. Relief of fibromyalgia symptoms following discontinuation of dietary excitotoxins. *Annals of Pharmocotherapy* 2001 Jun;35(6):702–6.

Sprott, H., et al. Microcirculatory changes over the tender points in fibromyalgia patients after acupuncture therapy (measured with laser-Doppler flowmetry). *Wiener Klinische Wochenschrift* 2000 Jul 7;112(13):580–6.

Szabo, A., et al. Phenylethylamine, a possible link to the antidepressant effects of exercise? *British Journal of Sports Medicine* 2001 Oct;35(5):342–3.

Tfelt-Hansen, P., Saxena, P.R., Dahlof, C., et al. Ergotamine in the acute treatment of migraine: a review and European consensus. *Brain* 2000; 123 (Pt 1):9.

Tuchin, P.J., et al. A Randomized Controlled Trial of Chiropractic Spinal Manipulative Therapy for Migraine. *Journal of Manipulative and Physiological Therapeutics* (February 2000) 23(2), 91–5.

Vincent, K.R., et al. Resistance exercise and bone turnover in elderly men and women. *Medical Science in Sports and Exercise* 2002 Jan;34(1):17–23.

Wilson, M.L. and Murphy, P.A. Herbal and dietary therapies for primary and secondary dysmenorrhoea. *Cochrane Database of Systematic Reviews.* 2001.

Yoshida, T., et al. Non-invasive measurement of brain activity using functional MRI: toward the study of brain response to acupuncture stimulation. *American Journal of Chinese Medicine*, 1995, 23(3–4):319–25.

Yunus, M.B., et al. Relationship between body mass index and fibromyalgia features. *Scandinavian Journal of Rheumatology* 2002;31(1):27–31.

Index